FLAWLESS

For Mum and Dad
For teaching me to dream boldly, work hard and always be kind.

MIX
Paper | Supporting responsible forestry
FSC® C011124
FSC www.fsc.org

First published in Great Britain in 2026
by Hamlyn, an imprint of
Octopus Publishing Group Ltd
Carmelite House
50 Victoria Embankment
London EC4Y 0DZ
www.octopusbooks.co.uk

An Hachette UK Company
www.hachette.co.uk

The authorized representative in the EEA is Hachette Ireland, 8 Castlecourt Centre, Dublin 15, D15 XTP3, Ireland (email: info@hbgi.ie)

Distributed in the US by Hachette Book Group, 1290 Avenue of the Americas, 4th and 5th Floors, New York NY 10104

Distributed in Canada by Canadian Manda Group, 664 Annette St, Toronto, Ontario, Canada M6S 2C8

ISBN: 978-0-600-64002-8
eISBN: 978-0-600-64003-5

A CIP catalogue record for this book is available from the British Library.

Printed and bound in Germany.

10 9 8 7 6 5 4 3 2 1

Publisher: Kate Fox
Art Director: Juliette Norsworthy
Senior Developmental Editor: Pauline Bache
Senior Editor: Leanne Bryan
Copyeditor: Emily Preece-Morrison
Project Editor: Emma Bastow
Designer: Clare Sivell
Illustrator: Claire Rollet
Production Manager: Nic Jones
Assistant Production Manager: Lucy Carter

Picture credits
Alamy: Scott Camazine 65r; iStock: bluecinema 47r, Cunaplus_M.Faba 65c, Ivanna Oliinyk 125, Janis Abolins 65l, LightFieldStudios 47l, Marina Demeshko 62, Olga Shefer 52, 55, samsonovs 4, Tatiana Foxy 58l; Shutterstock: Moteelec 59, New Africa 58r

FLAWLESS

Your ultimate guide to bright, clear skin

DR SAM BUNTING

hamlyn

CONTENTS

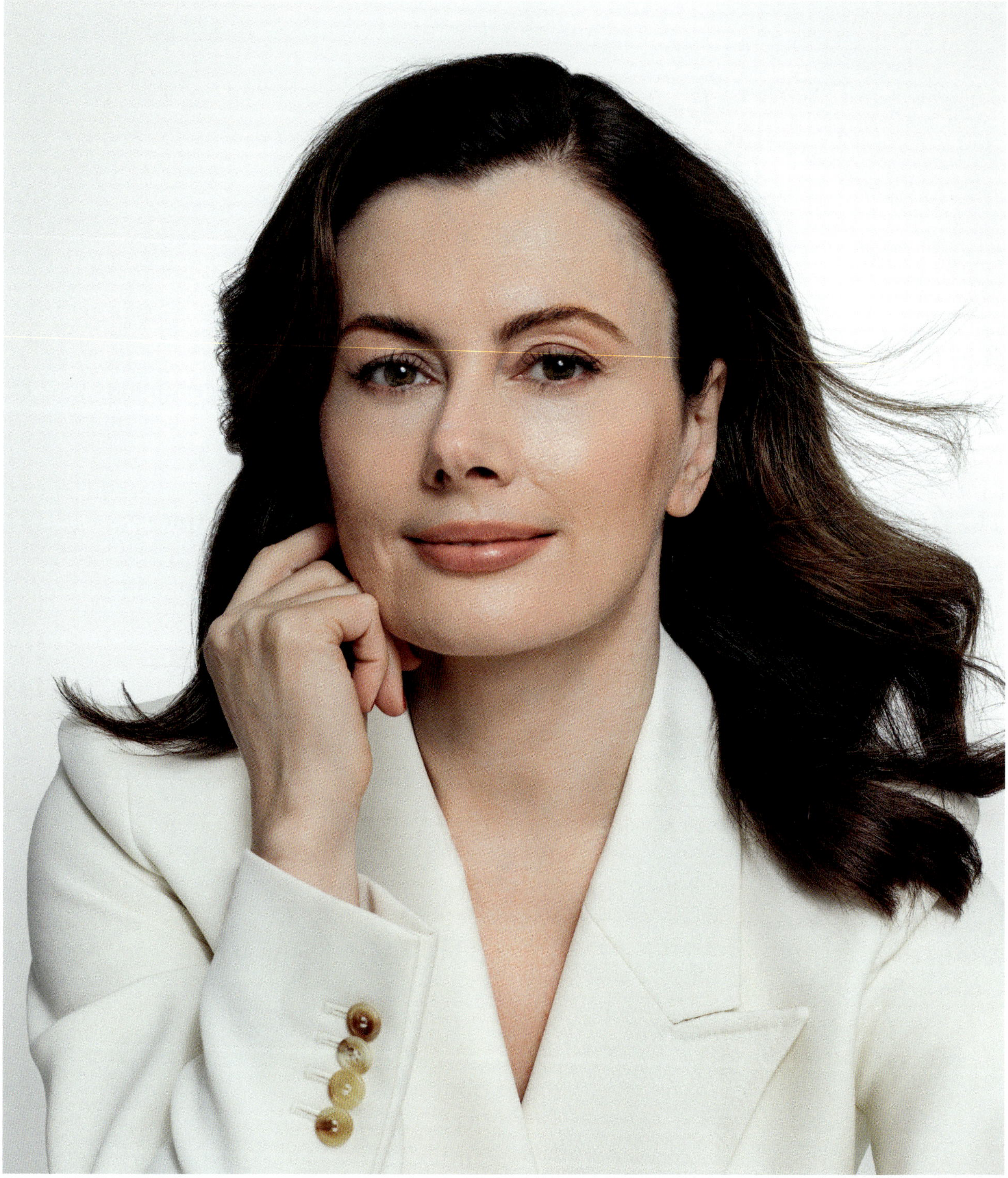

YOUR JOURNEY TO GREAT SKIN

I am Dr Sam Bunting, a cosmetic dermatologist specializing, quite simply, in great skin. I have spent two decades helping patients, followers and customers achieve the skin of their dreams.

I'm the founder of a Harley Street cosmetic dermatology clinic, and the founder of the award-winning Dr Sam's Skincare range. My entire career has been dedicated to making expert skincare advice more accessible and great skin more achievable. This book is the culmination of that journey and my philosophy distilled. In your hands you have a manual and catalyst for change, which I hope you'll find both practical and empowering, inspiring and transformative.

WHY DO WE CARE SO MUCH ABOUT OUR SKIN?

I can say with absolute conviction that the desire for good skin is hardwired into us as humans. Our skin health is a kind of shorthand for our internal health and genetic fitness. And it really is worth putting in the work. When you change your skin, it's no exaggeration to say you change your life. Having helped thousands of people embark on just such a journey over twenty years, I'm here to tell you that everyone can improve their skin and reap the immeasurable benefits: better skin, better health, more confidence, more freedom.

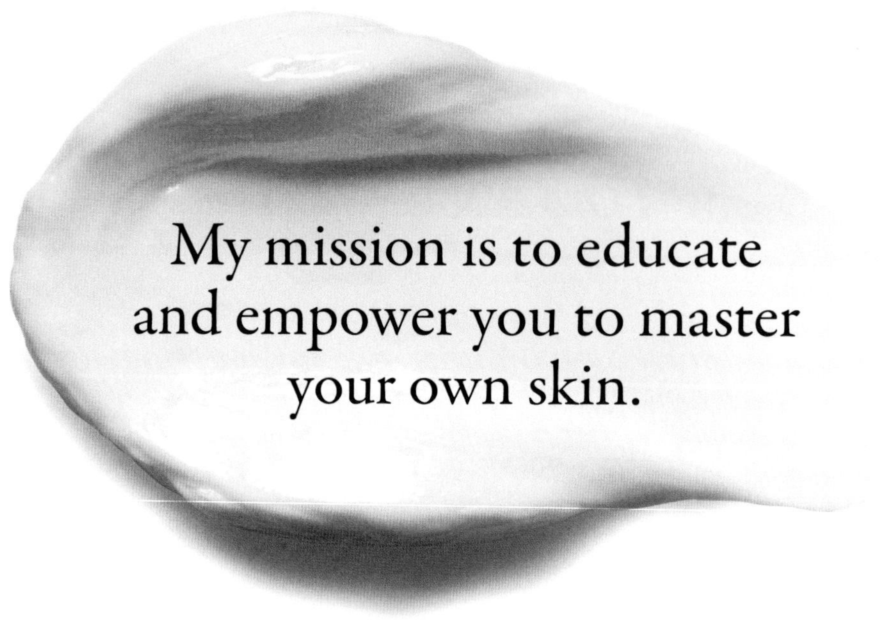

My mission is to educate and empower you to master your own skin.

But where do you go to find out what you should use on your skin? The words 'complex' and 'confusion' abound. We no longer seem to seek advice from our mums or magazines; instead, we've turned to the behemoth that is TikTok to tell us what products we need. The consequences of that can be catastrophic, especially if you have problem skin. Trending skincare does not mean it's skincare that's right for you. That's why I had to write this book – to help you develop mastery of *your* skin. Because it really doesn't have to be that hard.

WHY SHOULD YOU LISTEN TO ME?

I was obsessed with beauty before I was even a teenager, but when I studied Medicine at Cambridge University and beyond, I found myself fascinated by skincare. A bright, clear and predictable complexion was the Holy Grail. My own skin was a mess – study stress made me break out, and the breakouts made me stressed. I felt out of control with my skin. During my third year I got to study Pharmacology, which is when I fell head over heels for the science of drugs – their effects on living systems generally and their potential for skin transformation in particular. After graduation, while I was working as a junior doctor in Australia, where I saw the devastating impact of powerful and relentless UV exposure, I knew skin was going to be my thing.

Dermatology training beckoned. Alas, skincare and cosmetics were less of a focus in the UK, and it became clear to me that I wanted to practise in the way that was popular in the US, where the focus was on both medical and cosmetic dermatology. So, I took the plunge and started my own practice, doing things my way. I became known for a specific methodology: highly edited skincare recommendations, based on credible science and proven results, with a detailed and holistic approach. Word spread. Supermodels, Oscar-winning actresses and politicians all made their way to the clinic to book an appointment with me and get prescribed one of these protocols.

Thank goodness, skincare has changed a lot in the last ten years, and nowadays we have easy access to remarkable tools and ingredients previously only available to the privileged clientele of expensive doctors. But the problem is that much of the language around skincare relates to it as a beauty ritual, rather than something more scientific. As I often tell patients: skincare is not entertainment. But before you switch off and switch on your LED mask in a huff, that doesn't mean we can't have fun with it! It's just that fun shouldn't be our primary goal. I want you to get pleasure from the results, as well as the process.

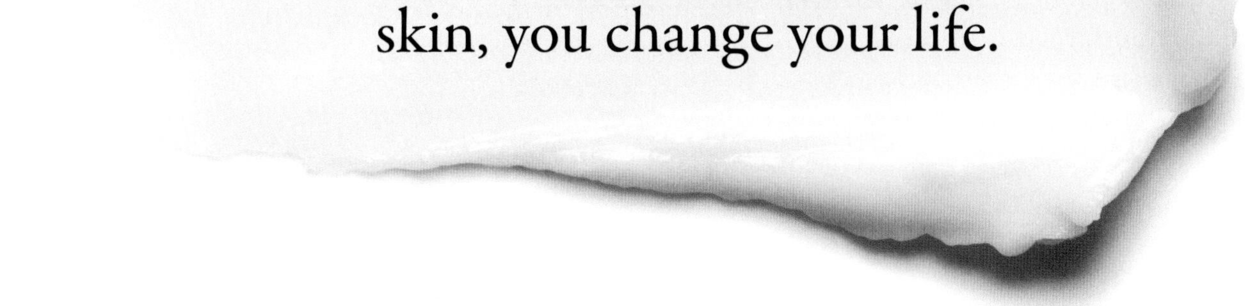

When you change your skin, you change your life.

MAKING SKINCARE SIMPLE

I think the modern framing of skincare as a consumer pursuit rather than a health practice is over-complex and the root cause of why so many of us feel confused, aimless and helpless. It has become increasingly difficult to navigate the daunting world of skincare without a compass. As a cosmetic dermatologist, I sit at the intersection of both worlds, and I feel the tension every single day. My job is to bring the rigour of medicine to a space that doesn't always welcome it. To ask the questions a good clinician always asks: 'What is the evidence?' 'What is the mechanism?' 'What are the risks?'

There's so much choice and conflicting advice; so many different brands and products, all promising skin nirvana. Hopes have been dashed, elixirs have overpromised and underdelivered, and if you're struggling with your skin, all you want is a solution. The problem is you can spend a lot of time, and hundreds of pounds, on the wrong thing. I launched Dr Sam's with one product – my Flawless Cleanser – and nothing else, because I wanted to help people get back to basics; strip out the noise, strip back their skincare regimes and rebuild with fewer products for maximum impact.

The idea of creating my own skincare range took root many years ago. I was always aware that not everyone with problem skin would be able to seek an appointment with a dermatologist. I also believe that, while we can't all have Angelina's lips or Kate Moss's cheekbones, everyone *can* aspire to great skin. The ways in which Dr Sam's is different to the rest of the market stems from our philosophy; the same philosophy that powers the clinic, the same philosophy that this book is built on: **simplicity, excellent advice and transformative skincare**.

HOW WILL THIS WORK FOR YOU?

I should point out that FLAWLESS isn't about achieving perfect skin. It's about using an approach for your skin that's flawless. In essence, I want it to be a complete end-to-end solution for your skin.

This book is where medical and cosmetic dermatology meet. It's not about whether to get filler or Botox, and it's not a science textbook. It's a colourful, practical, one-stop shop that will help you understand your skin, understand the products available, and create a bespoke skincare routine with confidence.

On my website, you can take a simple quiz, the Routine Finder, and receive a curated list of products and a plan to help you with your skin concerns. An easy experience from start to finish, it was designed to make you feel like you'd had a consultation with me in person. I also support it with video content as though I'm with you in your bathroom, coaching you to use your new routine, so there is zero guesswork. I am bringing exactly that philosophy and formula to you in this book, so you too can build a FLAWLESS routine based on the founding principles of my skin philosophy.

Whatever stage of life you're at, this book will give you a framework to start and maintain productive habits and practices that will optimize your skin health and appearance in the long-term. You will come away empowered, committed and confident. It's a self-help book for your skin, if you will. It's the book I wish had existed when I was looking for answers.

So, let's begin.

Dr Sam Bunting

1

The Dr Sam's Philosophy

IT DOESN'T HAVE TO BE COMPLICATED

There's a great line in the hit American TV show Seinfeld *from George Costanza after Jerry starts dating a dermatologist: 'Skin doesn't need a doctor; wash it, dry it, move on!'*

George, you're a hoot, but it's a teensy bit more complicated than that. I'm hoping that once you've finished this book, you'll feel as confident in mastering skincare as George is at dismissing it. I'll start by letting you in on the secrets of my philosophy: the principles I use for my own skin, my practice, my brand. This is Dr Sam, barefaced.

I am deeply, uncompromisingly rational about skincare. And while skincare requires more than George would have us believe, it doesn't have to be as complicated as much of the beauty industry portrays it. We're in the midst of an epidemic of inflammatory skin issues such as adult acne and perioral dermatitis, another common and annoying acne-like disorder of the skin (more on this later), and I think that many fashionable modern skincare practices have played a role in that. You don't need a ten-step skincare routine. My patients are often staggered that something as simple as a product cull can rapidly help bring their issues under control. 'Less is more' has never been truer when it comes to our skin. If a product, procedure or practice is making a move on your routine, you need an excellent reason for it to be there. My rule is: if you want to be on my face, you need to earn your place!

As the philosopher Will Durant said: 'we are what we repeatedly do'. Our daily habits have the power to define us – and when it comes to a daily skincare routine, consistency can deliver remarkable results. Thanks to the principle of marginal gains, small incremental changes can add up to significant improvements over time, if you keep at it. It may feel hard to begin and commit to new skincare practices – even if they're less elaborate than your old ones – but once you're in the swing of things, you'll fall in love with the process and the results will take care of themselves.

Looking after your skin can be both relaxing and rewarding, but it's easy to become trapped in an expensive and overcomplicated hobby for the sake of it. Buy and use what YOU need to get the job done. You'll save time and money, and feel freer. Think about incorporating these ideas into your routine and you'll be the master of your skin – not the other way around.

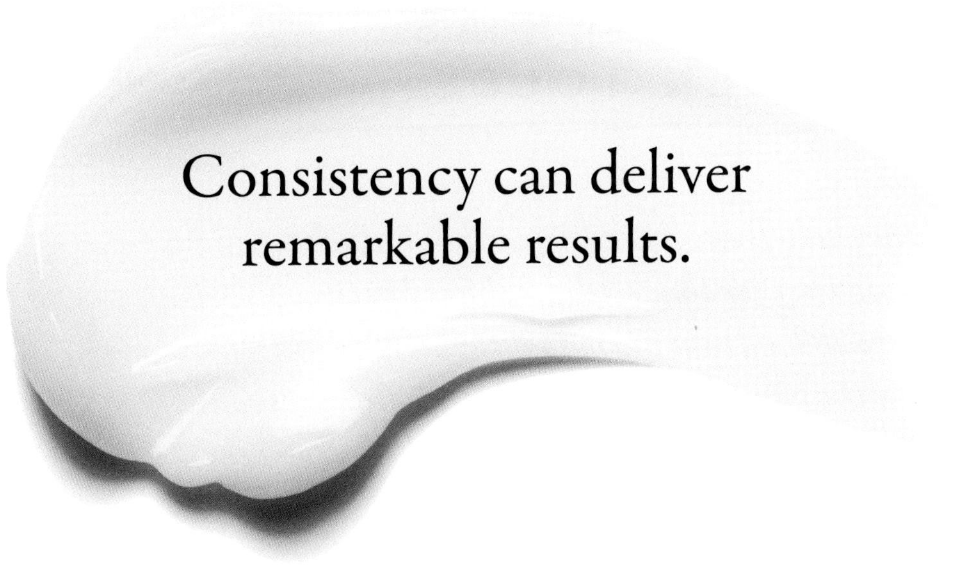

Consistency can deliver remarkable results.

DR SAM'S SKINCARE PHILOSOPHY

- **Keep it simple**
  Fewer steps = better results.
- **Do no harm**
  Every product has to earn its place.
  If it irritates or overcomplicates, bin it.
- **Consistency beats intensity**
  Daily habits, stacked up over time, deliver real results.
- **Skin is rational**
  Treat it with logic, evidence and restraint, not myths, hype or quick fixes.
- **Control what you can**
  Throw energy at things you can influence and make peace with things you can't.
- **Fall in love with the process**
  Skincare should feel rewarding, not confusing.

TEN THINGS THAT DON'T MATTER AS MUCH AS YOU'VE BEEN TOLD

A lot of beauty beliefs are passed on without much interrogation, whether that's advice shared between friends, passed down from mum to daughter, or indeed gleaned from the pages of glossy magazines. But we should be more questioning of the origins of these diktats, since many are simply outdated or works of fiction. Here is a sample of beliefs and practices that I have little use for when building protocols for my patients.

1 DRINKING WATER

Beauty lore cites drinking water (eight glasses a day, specifically) as the cure for everything from acne to dull, dehydrated skin.

Alas, water has no ability to flush out the toxins of acne (there aren't any) and unless you address your skin barrier health, any extra water that makes its way to your skin will simply evaporate away. Drink enough for your general health and your skin will be fine.

2 SILK PILLOWCASES

These feel nice. However, when it comes to wrinkles, the weight of the human head is the problem. It's around 5kg (11lb), so when you sleep on your side or on your front, that's a heavy weight squishing the skin of your face for around seven hours a night, creating those etched-in sleep lines. Every day, for years . . . No fine material can mitigate that, unfortunately. Training yourself to sleep on your back is the answer.

3 TONERS

Once upon a time, we used actual soap to cleanse our skin. However, the nature of soap is that it's alkaline and leaves a residue behind that disrupts the skin's mildly acidic pH (known as the acid mantle). This can damage our skin barrier, so liquid toners were developed to get rid of this residue and restore the skin's pH back to a healthy level.

These days, cleansers are an entirely different beast – they are pH balanced and rinse clear. So, modern toners have been reinvented – they now deliver ingredients one might like to leave behind, such as an exfoliating acid, for example.

I believe that we should be more intentional when applying ingredients to our skin and use measured amounts of leave-on products, so we know what dose we are depositing on the skin. That's why I relegate toners to the bin of unnecessary products.

4 GENES

Many people think that having 'good genes' means you will have better skin. I'm going to play devil's advocate here . . . and say that genes don't really matter. When it comes to ageing, our genetic blueprint governs about 20 per cent of the process. That's it. At least 80 per cent of ageing is determined by what happens outside our bodies in the environment. This is such excellent news. It means that 80 per cent of how we age is within our control.

5 PHYSICAL EXFOLIATION

Your skin sheds its surface cells naturally, all by itself, every single day. Scrubs and brushes attempt to hurry this along in a quest for smoothness, but they're imprecise, often stripping away cells your skin still needs. That satisfying grit? It's doing more harm than good.

6 CELLULITE CREAMS

It's very hard to influence things that are due to essentially how we are made. Women's bodies are equipped with a fibrous network containing fat cells layered under the skin on our thighs and hips. A bit like in a well-worn mattress, the fat eventually wants to poke out. Whether you are voluptuous or slender, that is the nature of this fat. It's why almost all women have some degree of cellulite. It's completely normal. No cream can reach this layer (nor should it – that would be dangerous), which is why cellulite creams don't work.

7 ANY HOME DEVICE THAT CLAIMS TO LIFT YOUR FACE

So seductive. But alas, anything that claims to lift is likely to be appealing to your hopes and dreams, and is probably going to leave them dashed. Lifting the skin without surgery is very hard, even within the confines of the doctor's office.

These home devices have very little power and, most importantly, can't make damaged elastin, our skin's built-in spring, regain its recoil.

This is the golden rule of elastin – you need to protect what you've got, because you can't rebuild it when it's gone. Elastin makes up only around 4 per cent of the protein in our skin (we have much more collagen), but once we reach puberty, we have received our lot.

8 STRETCH-MARK CREAMS

Stretch marks are tears in the elastin fibres in the skin over areas like the stomach, hips and thighs. During a teenage growth spurt or pregnancy, rapid stretching leads to these tears. Again, I counsel patients that these are so common as to be normal, so save your money when it comes to stretch-mark creams.

9 THOSE SEXY LITTLE GUA SHAS AND JADE ROLLERS

Sigh. Another practice that many people enjoy as part of a self-care ritual. No bad thing, but they won't sculpt a jawline or cheekbones, as many influencers promise. If you are prone to a little fluid retention, this might help clear it, but that's about it. The skin has an excellent blood supply so these will probably do no better job than going for a run.

10 FACIALS

When people hear I don't believe in facials, they often look as though I've told them there's no Father Christmas. The thing with facials is managing expectations. If you have a problem like acne or rosacea, there's a good chance you are at risk of making your problem worse with a facial. Inflammatory skin conditions do not like episodic pulses of new products; they like consistent application of correctly chosen ones that tackle the issues at their root cause. The friction from facial massage isn't a great idea either when dealing with inflammatory skin issues.

Ultimately, little can be achieved by a monthly facial that can't be done more effectively in a slow, steady and intentional way with the correct active ingredients administered by your own hands.

Of course, for some, facials are part of their self-care habits and that's great, as long as they do no harm. But if you want to be pampered, I'd rather you enjoyed a massage.

FIVE THINGS THAT MATTER MORE THAN YOU THINK

I hope I've convinced you that George was wrong – that skin does *need more than washing and drying. I'm here to coach you in the practices and products I believe are worth your time. Because life is better with bright, clear skin.*

1 DAILY SUNSCREEN USE

The simple act of wearing daily sunscreen is probably the most powerful thing you will ever do for your skin.

Eighty per cent of skin ageing is a result of environmental damage, most of which is caused by UV radiation from the sun. My philosophy is that the best sunscreen is the one you enjoy using. If I can convince you to start including SPF in your daily routine and never miss it (even if you're home sick with the flu), this one habit will change your skin. (More on this on pages 83–7 and 130–1.)

2 DO NO HARM WHEN YOU CLEANSE

If you get cleansing wrong, it's hard to get skincare right. Too often, I have seen first-hand the carnage overly elaborate cleansing routines can cause. Oil cleansers, double cleansing, assisted cleansing with vibrating brushes . . . it's all unnecessary.

Cleansing is the perfect example of why simplicity rules in skincare. You want to use the least irritating and barrier-depleting product to get off what needs to come off (dead skin cells, oil, make-up and SPF). That's it. That's all we should ask of a cleanser. It can't solve issues like acne. It can't cook you dinner. It can only clean your face.

3

DON'T BE AFRAID OF RETINOIDS

Too many people have walked away from retinoids, thinking they're not for them and this is almost always a mistake.

This scary word elicits foreboding in even some of the most seasoned beauty journalists, but in my chapter on Demystifying Active Ingredients (pages 89–119), I will show you how to use them correctly and safely.

4

BEAUTIFUL SKIN IS HYDRATED SKIN

Moisturizers are the largest skincare category. I think most people have an idea of what they're supposed to do, but not whether they're using a moisturizer that actually suits their skin. It's so important to get this step right, because it's the gateway to using actives, and actives are where the magic lies (see Demystifying Active Ingredients, pages 89–119).

5

STRESS DOES AFFECT OUR SKIN

We humans are excellent at not dealing with stress – we suppress it, override it and carry on. Can you guess where those bottled-up emotions often declare themselves? Correct: our skin. Our skin and our nervous system are inextricably intertwined. So when your mind is overwhelmed, your skin frequently tells the tale, something anyone with eczema or acne will confirm.

Personally, I have found incredible relief in Vedic meditation, cold-water therapy and a large glass of very good red beside a fire with a true friend, and a cat on my lap.

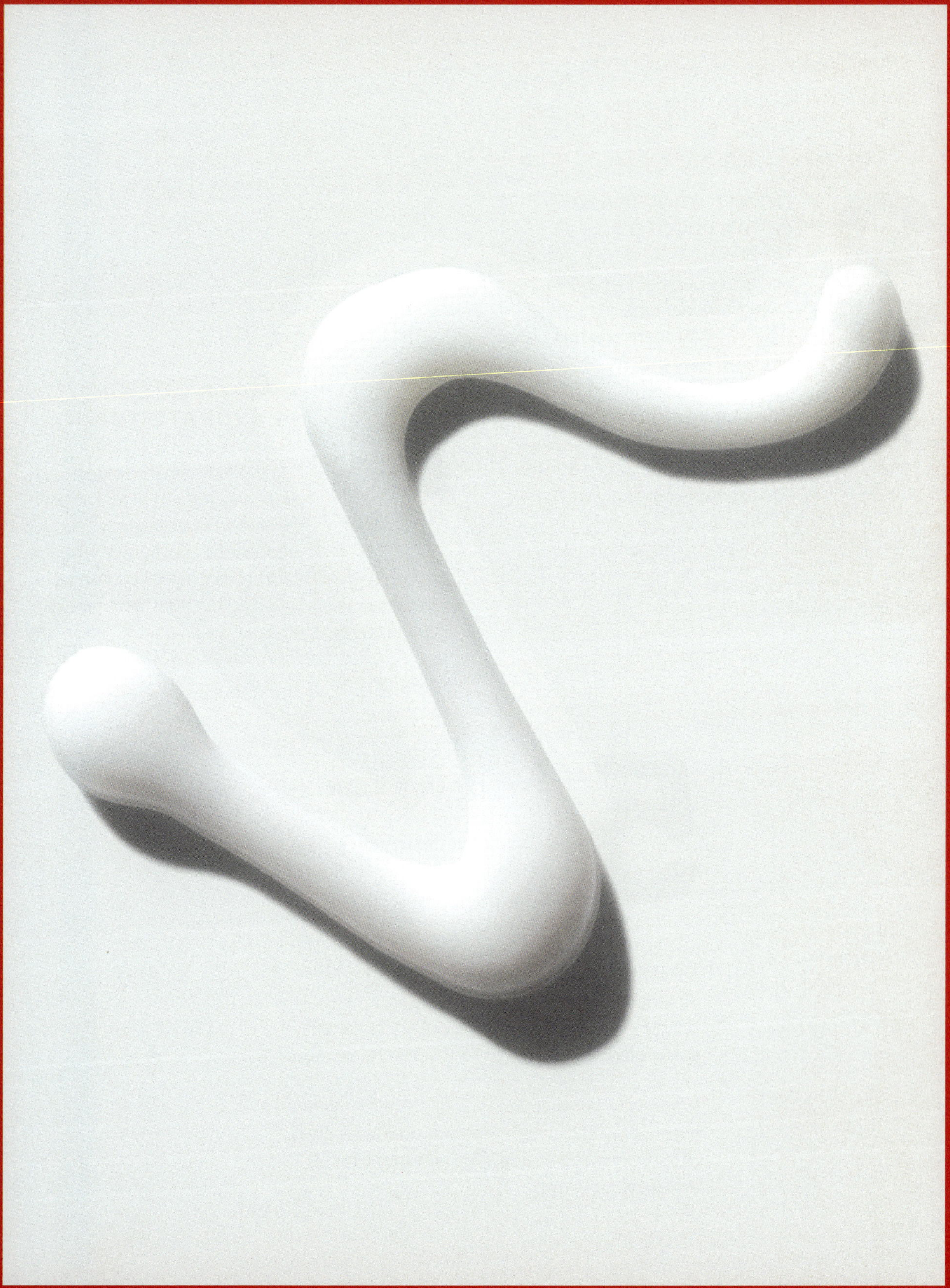

2

Skin 101

INTRODUCING YOUR SKIN

Skin is fabulous stuff. It's our wrapper – the interface that connects our insides with the outside world.

It forms an external tube that connects directly with our internal one – the gut. It's a mind-bogglingly active organ, not some passive structure. We might be able to visualize this action more easily with an organ like our heart, but our skin is just as busy.

For this book, we will focus our interest on the two outermost layers of the skin – the epidermis and dermis – because, when it comes to skincare, these are the layers we can influence.

But first: a smidgeon of anatomy. I'm going to take you on a whistle-stop tour of your skin so that you can understand its structure, function and behaviour, because I believe that demystifying the science of skin will help you make better choices when it comes to skin care.

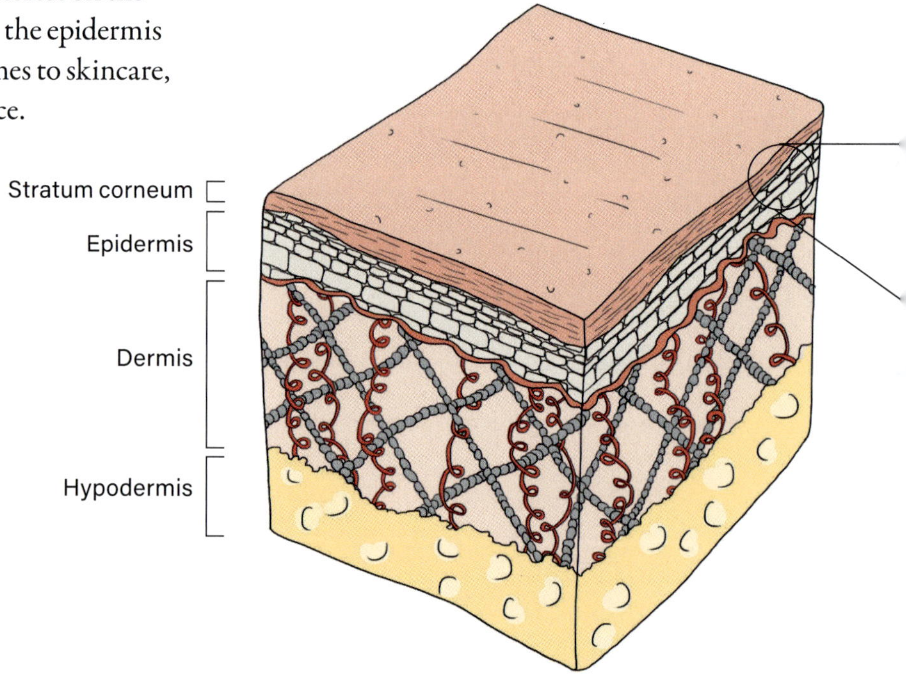

THE SKIN STRUCTURE

THE SKIN BARRIER

You might be inclined to think of the epidermis as a passive raincoat, shielding us from our environment. But when you zoom in, it's anything but.

Protection comes from the outermost part of the epidermis, in a structure called the stratum corneum. Commonly known as the 'skin barrier', the stratum corneum can be thought of as a wall. Its cells form a structure similar to bricks and mortar. How well maintained that wall is determines much of how our skin looks and feels, and how good it is at keeping the bad stuff out.

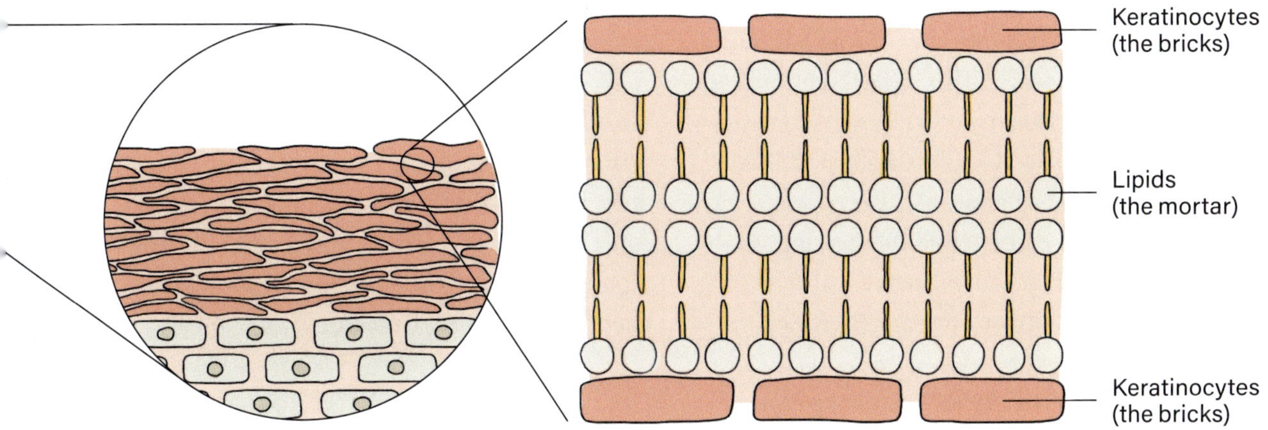

THE STRATUM CORNEUM

The bricks in our wall are skin cells, known as keratinocytes. By the time they reach the stratum corneum, they've undergone a remarkable transformation. Starting life in the deepest layer of the epidermis, they gradually flatten, fill with a tough protein called keratin, release their fats – which form the mortar around the bricks – and eventually die. What arrives at the skin's surface is a purpose-built defence unit: a tough cell packed with keratin and water-binding substances called Natural Moisturizing Factor (NMF), wrapped in a shell of proteins and lipids. This is what your skin barrier is actually made of.

The wall is typically around 15 cell layers deep in white skin and up to 20 layers thick in darker skin tones. It can be even thicker in areas that need more protection, such as the hands and feet.

The integrity of this wall is so important that our body replaces it constantly. This replacement takes roughly 28 days. The stratum corneum itself turns over faster, being replaced every couple of weeks in a process called 'desquamation'. The process is invisible, constant and essential. When it goes wrong or slows down, it can be seen as dullness or roughness of the skin, or uneven skin tone.

The mortar between the bricks is made up of a structured mix of lipids: ceramides, cholesterol and fatty acids, arranged in precise layers. These form a seal that locks water and nutrients in. They also hold the cells together in an organized structure that keeps the skin barrier intact.

Inside each brick, the NMF, a blend of amino acids, urea and other small molecules, pulls water into the cell and holds it there. If the mortar keeps things sealed, the NMF keeps each cell plump and hydrated. Together they are the reason your skin holds onto water at all, and why it feels dry when either element is depleted.

Not all skin builds the same wall. In fact, darker skin produces lower levels of the lipids called ceramides, which are crucial for locking in moisture. This creates a paradox: a physically thicker wall that can nonetheless lose moisture more easily and behave more reactively.

Along the way, keratinocytes also produce antioxidants that help neutralize free radicals triggered by UV exposure and pollution. And the epidermis is where melanin and vitamin D are produced.

The stratum corneum is proof that the body's most brilliant innovations are often its most invisible ones. In its precisely ordered architecture, its constant cycle of renewal, and its extraordinary capacity to adapt, the skin barrier stands as a masterpiece of human biology.

THE MICROBIOME

Now, it's time to meet the residents. Living on top of your skin barrier is a vast community of bacteria, viruses and yeasts, collectively known as the microbiome.

To give you a sense of scale: the microbial DNA on your skin outnumbers your own human DNA by 100 to 300 times. Far from being unwanted passengers, the microbiome is a core part of your skin's defences. It helps train your immune system, dampen inflammation and fight off harmful bacteria that might otherwise colonize the surface.

These residents vary from place to place on your body. The community on your face is quite different to the one in your armpit. And it shifts over time: the microbiome you had during puberty won't be the one you carry through menopause. These shifts influence everything from skin diseases like acne and eczema, to how your skin ages.

The microbiome on the surface of your skin is fussy about pH. The surface of your skin sits at a pH of around 4.7, which is slightly acidic, thanks to a mix of sweat, sebum and byproducts released by our keratinocytes as they reach the end of their life cycle. This natural defence film, known as the 'acid mantle', creates an environment where beneficial microbes thrive and harmful ones struggle to take hold.

What makes all of this remarkable is that the barrier and the microbiome aren't separate systems – they regulate each other. The barrier's pH supports the right microbial balance. The microbiome, in turn, reinforces the barrier. Disrupt one and you destabilize both. This is why something as simple as cleansing matters far more than you might think. It's not surface-level care. It's ecosystem maintenance.

AT A GLANCE: THE ACID MANTLE

What it is: A thin, acidic film (pH ~4.7) made of sweat, sebum and skin cell byproducts.

What it does: Keeps skin hydrated, defends against microbes, supports the microbiome.

Why it matters: Disrupted mantle = dryness, irritation, skin more prone to inflammation and infection.

THE PIGMENT SYSTEM

Now, let's go deeper and home in on a very important cell at the bottom of the epidermis – the melanocyte.

This is the source of your skin pigment, known as melanin. It is your natural sunscreen.

UV (ultraviolet) radiation is the invisible electromagnetic radiation emitted by the sun's rays and used in tanning beds. It is categorized into UVA, UVB and UVC wavelengths. While UVC is blocked by the ozone layer and doesn't reach Earth, UVA and UVB radiation do penetrate the skin, get absorbed and cause damage.

The purpose of the pigment system is to patrol and protect the health of the DNA housed in the nucleus of the keratinocyte stem cells at the bottom of the epidermis. Think of it as your skin's UV neighbourhood watch. These special keratinocytes serve as a reservoir and are dividing constantly to replace the ones being lost at the skin's surface, so their DNA is vulnerable and precious, and its integrity must be protected at all costs.

When there's a threat to your skin (such as a midday lunch outdoors in summer when you've forgotten to apply sunscreen), the DNA inside your keratinocytes gets zapped by the sun's UVB rays and this damage activates the melanocytes. Your melanocytes spring into action, each delivering protection to shield around 30 keratinocytes. The melanocytes unload melanin packaged in parcels called melanosomes into each of these keratinocytes. The melanin then sits on

THE SPECTRUM OF UV EFFECTS

UVB (5% of UV): Burns, directly damages DNA, drives skin cancer. Triggers melanin production leading to delayed tanning.

UVA (95% of UV): Penetrates deeper, does indirect damage via oxidative stress (see page 40), causing ageing and increased risk of skin cancer. As it oxidizes existing melanin it can cause an immediate tan.

UVC: Blocked by ozone, so it doesn't reach Earth.

What this means: Daily broad-spectrum SPF is non-negotiable.

1 Melanocytes are stimulated by UV light.
2 Melanin pigment is produced inside melanosomes.
3 Melanosomes are transferred to keratinocyte cells.
4 Melanin is removed when the dead skin cells are shed.

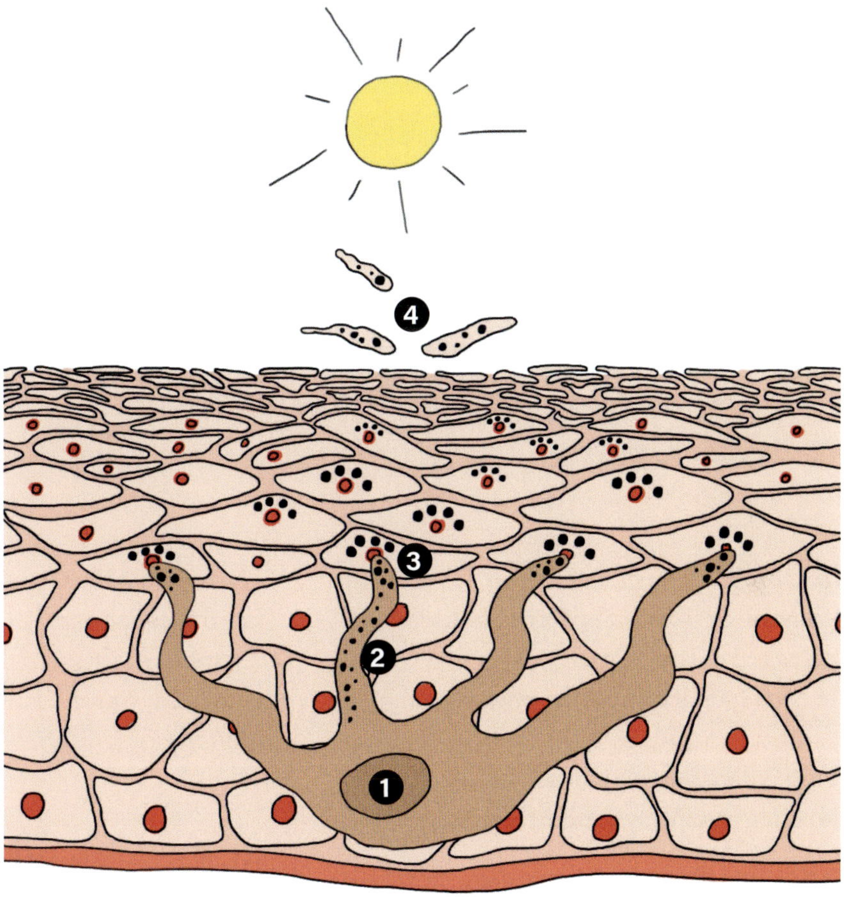

THE MELANOCYTE/KERATINOCYTE INTERACTION WHEN WE TAN

top of their nucleus, like a parasol, and absorbs the UVB rays before they can damage any more DNA.

This all takes a bit of time. After a couple of days, it causes the skin to develop what we know as a tan. When you appreciate that this is a response to UV radiation *directly* damaging chemical bonds in your skin's DNA, you can understand why there's no such thing as a safe tan.

During that sunny lunch, you're also exposed to UVA rays. While these are lower energy than UVB rays and don't directly damage DNA, they create unstable molecules called reactive oxygen species (ROS; see page 40 for more on these) and trigger oxidation of melanin that's been prepared earlier by your melanocytes, which is already inside your keratinocytes. Melanin that's become oxidized immediately darkens.

Our natural UV defences do their best, but they're imperfect and outdated. They evolved for survival, not to preserve skin health across the many decades we now live. Don't rely on them alone when smart sun habits and daily sunscreen can do what nature never intended: keep skin truly healthy for life.

DECONSTRUCTING YOUR SKIN TONE

What determines your skin colour isn't the number of melanocytes you have.

We all have roughly the same number. It's what the melanosomes look like and how they behave once they're delivered to your keratinocytes that counts. There are two types of melanin pigment:

Eumelanin is dark brown or black and acts like a sponge, soaking up UV rays before they can do harm.

Pheomelanin is a lighter, reddish-yellow pigment that absorbs very little UV and offers far less protection. We're all born with the ability to make both pigments. It's the ratio your genes dial up or down that shapes your natural skin tone.

But it's not just about the type of melanin. In lighter skin, melanosomes are small, bundled together in clusters, and broken down quickly as keratinocytes move towards the surface. In darker skin, they're larger, individually dispersed, and persist much further up through the epidermis. This is why darker skin offers significantly more natural UV protection (see table, opposite).

There is one final thing to mention about these clever cells: your melanocytes can actually sense visible light, helping skin get in tune with your circadian rhythms (your internal body clock). They use proteins called opsins to detect high-energy blue light, just like your eyes do. When stimulated, your melanocytes shift gear and produce more melanin.

THE MELANIN MISFIRE

Melanocytes don't just patrol for sun damage – they're on high alert for any local disturbance. Inflammation triggered by injury, irritation or skin disease releases chemical messengers that signal stress in the area. In response, melanocytes may ramp up melanin production or redistribute pigment, often unevenly. This creates what's known as post-inflammatory hyperpigmentation (PIH).

This is an evolutionary mismatch; a system built to respond to UV threat gets activated by inflammation too, producing pigment where none is needed. In darker skin, where melanosomes are larger, individually dispersed and persist further through the epidermis, the response is more pronounced and slower to resolve. The same characteristics that give darker skin superior UV protection also make it more vulnerable to visible pigmentary fallout from even minor disruption. This is why so much of what we'll cover later, from sunscreen to managing inflammation, is grounded in keeping your pigment system steady.

THE FITZPATRICK PHOTOTYPING SYSTEM

Developed by dermatologist Thomas Fitzpatrick in 1975, this system classifies skin into six types based on how it responds to UV exposure. It's a useful clinical shorthand, not just for predicting burn risk, but for understanding why darker skin types are more prone to pigmentary fallout from inflammation, and why SPF recommendations aren't one-size-fits-all.

SKIN TYPE		
TYPE I		**PALE WHITE SKIN** *extremely sensitive skin, always burns, never tans* Example: Red hair with freckles
TYPE II		**WHITE SKIN** *very sensitive skin, burns easily, tans minimally* Example: Fair-skinned, fair-haired Caucasians, northern Asians
TYPE III		**LIGHT BROWN SKIN** *sensitive skin, sometimes burns, slowly tans to light brown* Example: Darker Caucasians, some Asians
TYPE IV		**MODERATE BROWN SKIN** *mildly sensitive, burns minimally, always tans to moderate brown* Example: Mediterranean and Middle Eastern Caucasians, southern Asians
TYPE V		**DARK BROWN SKIN** *resistant skin, rarely burns, tans well* Example: Some Hispanics, some Africans
TYPE VI		**DEEPLY PIGMENTED DARK BROWN TO BLACK SKIN** *very resistant skin, never burns, deeply pigmented* Example: Darker Africans, Indigenous Australians

THE HAIR FOLLICLE

The hair follicle is far more than a shaft for growing hair. It's a powerful ecosystem in its own right.

It houses sebaceous glands, hormone receptors and a two-way line of communication with the immune system. It's also where acne, one of the most common skin concerns, begins. Each hair follicle is a tunnel reaching from the dermis to its opening on the surface of your skin. This opening is called a pore. Just like the stratum corneum, the lining of the follicle is made up of keratinocytes

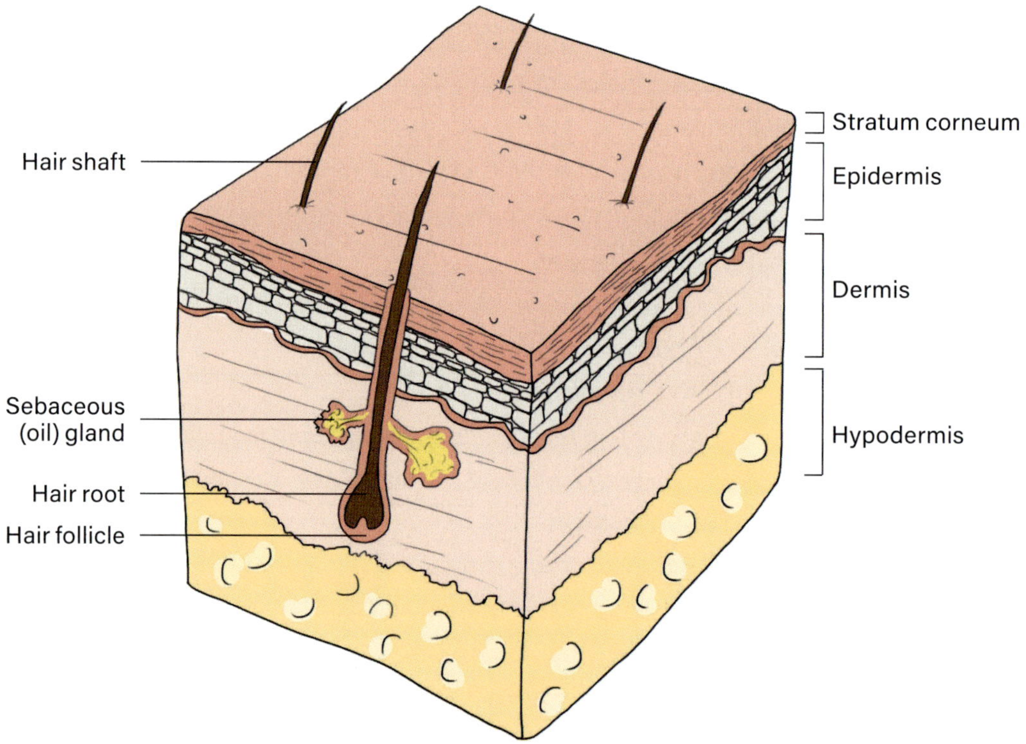

THE HAIR FOLLICLE STRUCTURE

which, under normal circumstances, shed in an orderly fashion, much like the desquamation happening on the skin's surface above.

Along the walls of the tunnel lie sebaceous glands, which produce sebum, a lipid-loaded, waxy substance that travels up the follicle, out of the pore and spreads across the skin's surface creating what we see as oil or shine. Sebum helps prevent water loss and contributes to the skin's acid mantle. Crucially, and contrary to popular belief, pores do not open and close like doors. Their size is influenced by several things: how much oil is flowing through them, your genetics, and cumulative sun damage over time. When everything is in balance, this is an elegant system.

Hair follicles also have receptors for hormonal messengers transmitted in our blood called androgens (like testosterone), which are found in both men and women, albeit at different levels. These messengers control how much sebum your skin makes, how fast hair grows and how easily the skin becomes inflamed.

During puberty, rising androgens cause sebaceous glands to shift up a gear, pumping out far more oil and making skin in the T-zone look shiny and the pores look bigger. They also make the follicle-lining keratinocytes sticky – instead of shedding cleanly, they start to clump together. This mixes with the extra oil and blocks pores, setting the stage for blackheads (open comedones), whiteheads (closed comedones) and their close cousin, acne.

The follicle is also home to much of your skin's microbiome, notably featuring bacteria called *Cutibacterium acnes* (*C. acnes*). Normally harmless, this species becomes problematic when a blocked follicle traps excess sebum, giving *C. acnes* lots to feast on. The bacteria break down the sebum's triglycerides into pro-inflammatory fatty acids, triggering an immune response. That's when you feel it: redness, swelling and a visible breakout.

In ideal conditions, the hair follicle is a friend, helping skin stay hydrated and connected to the wider hormonal and microbial network. At its worst, the follicle can become a site of real damage. In cases of cystic acne or persistent folliculitis, the environment becomes deeply inflamed, with immune cells flooding in and creating destruction that can linger as permanent scarring.

Where your follicles fall on that spectrum is influenced by your genetics, your hormones, your stress levels and, crucially, your skincare habits.

THE DERMIS: WHERE YOUTH LIES

Beneath all of this lies a sturdy yet dynamic infrastructure that keeps everything in place, providing vital support, strength and resilience.

That is the essence of your dermis and there is one critical cell you need to know about to understand the key to a youthful complexion: the fibroblast. The fibroblasts are the factories responsible for building your skin's foundations. They produce, assemble and maintain most of the critical structural elements that keep your skin bouncy, firm and robust. When you hear the word 'anti-ageing' in skincare, think fibroblast.

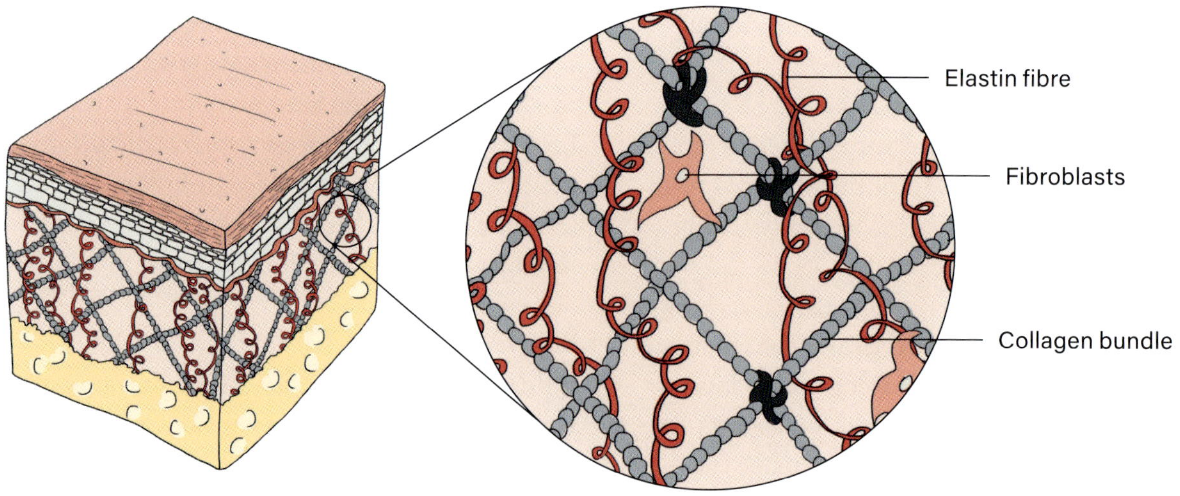

THE FIBROBLAST

COLLAGEN:
YOUR SKIN'S SUPPORT BEAMS

Fibroblasts manufacture collagen, the most plentiful protein in the body. Much of it lies in the skin, where it acts like steel beams, holding your skin firm and smooth. It's the most plentiful protein in the body and much of it lies in your skin. If you were to take all the water out of your skin, 80 per cent of what's left behind would be collagen.

Your collagen is constantly being remodelled, so that old collagen that has become frayed and ravaged gets efficiently replaced by perky new cells, maintaining the status quo.

However, as we age and expose our skin to environmental challenges such as the sun and pollution, the balance shifts. The systems that remove old, worn-out collagen ramp up, while those that replace it slow down. The result is a collagen deficit and what we see on the surface of the skin as wrinkles.

When it comes to wrinkle formation, the size of your dermis matters. Darker skin has the advantage here, as it tends to have a thicker dermis and more densely packed collagen, making it more resistant to the collagen-stealing consequences of the sun. The flipside of this is when skin repairs and forms a scar, with new collagen replacing damaged collagen, darker skin has a higher risk of bulky scars, known as hypertrophic or keloid scars. So, while the signs of ageing may be delayed, there's a greater need to handle skin gently to minimize trauma and prevent scarring.

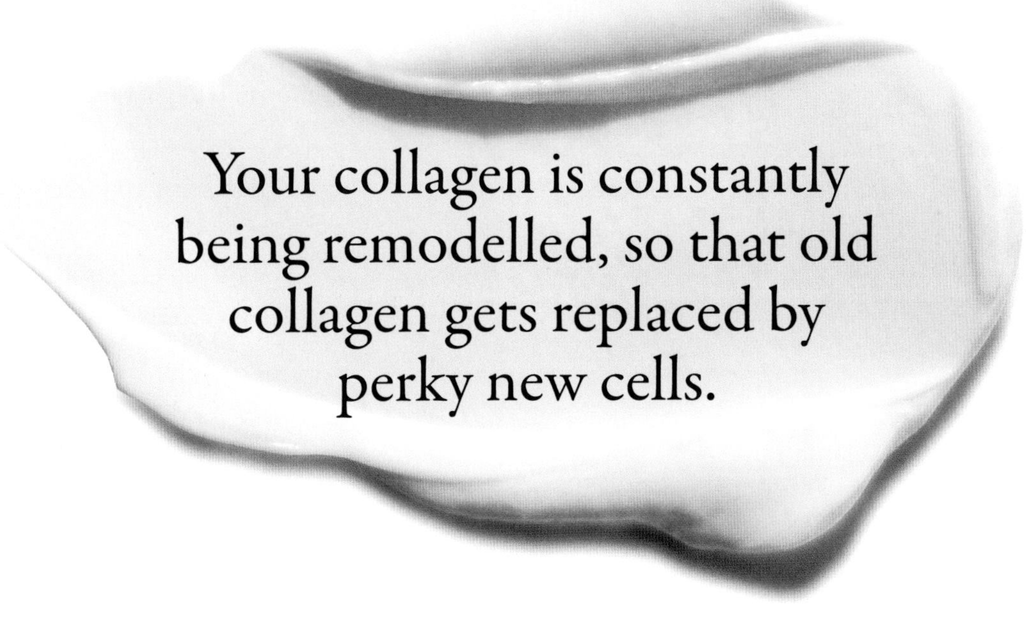

ELASTIN:
THE FLEXIBLE CABLES

Your fibroblasts bear a lot of responsibility, as they also produce elastin. Elastin is a protein that operates like springy cables in the skin, allowing it to stretch and then snap back into position, preventing sagging. In my opinion, elastin is not talked about enough in skincare. It's important to remember the golden rule of elastin: we need to protect what we've got, because we can't rebuild it to the same standard when it's gone. By contrast, collagen, which we can easily persuade our skin to make more of, tends to dominate the conversation.

The first place the loss of elastin tends to show up is in the ultra-thin skin of the eye area. When we smile, the skin beneath the eye is compressed under the squeezing force of the circular muscle that closes our eye (the orbicularis oculi). When the skin's elastin starts to deteriorate under the cumulative influence of UVA rays, this leads to a bunching effect, as the skin's snap isn't quite as good. I liken this to a vintage Alaïa Lycra dress losing its shape. Smoking and pollution also take their toll on your precious elastin.

HYALURONIC ACID AND GLYCOSAMINOGLYCANS:
THE DEEP HYDRATION SYSTEM

As if that wasn't enough, fibroblasts also produce the skin's internal hydration reservoirs. The most well known of these is hyaluronic acid (HA), a molecule made from repeating sugar units that can hold up to 1,000 times its weight in water. In the dermis, hyaluronic acid acts like a sponge, drawing water in and keeping the deeper layers of your skin plump and hydrated from within.

NOTES FROM THE CLINIC

Patients are often surprised when I tell them that their £200+ hyaluronic acid serum isn't going to turn back the clock. The hyaluronic acid in your serum and the hyaluronic acid in your dermis do very different jobs.

Topical HA molecules are too large to penetrate beyond the upper layers of the skin, so they hydrate the surface. The HA your fibroblasts produce works much deeper, maintaining the structural hydration that gives skin its volume. Dermal HA declines with age and no topical serum can replace it, but it can support the surface while you protect what lies beneath.

THE EYE AREA: A SPECIAL CASE

The skin around your eyes is not simply a thinner version of the skin covering the rest of your face: it's structurally distinct. This skin is roughly a third of the thickness of the skin covering your cheeks and contains fewer sebaceous glands, which means it has less natural lubrication and a barrier that dries out and breaks down more quickly.

This is also the hardest-working skin on your face; you blink around 20 times a minute, and every smile, squint and frown adds mechanical stress. This is why crow's feet and fine lines appear around the eye first, especially as elastin deteriorates. Beneath the surface, delicate fat pads and thinner connective tissue make this area prone to puffiness, hollowing and dark circles, where muscle and blood vessels show through simply because there's less skin covering them.

Because the skin around the eye is thinner, products penetrate more easily here, which sounds like a good thing until you realize it also means there's a higher risk of irritation. Ingredients that your cheeks tolerate comfortably can cause stinging and redness around the eyes.

All of this explains why the eye area needs its own skincare strategy – something we'll come to when we build your skincare routine (see pages 132–5).

The skin around your eyes is the hardest-working skin on your face.

OUR SKIN AND THE SUN

Perhaps the most important external relationship our skin has is with the sun.

The sun is essential to life. Its light powers the skin's production of vitamin D and helps set our internal clock, fine-tuning daily rhythms such as sleep and hormone release. However, sunlight is also a constant source of stress. Let's explore these roles, one by one.

When exposed to UVB rays, keratinocytes convert a cholesterol precursor into previtamin D3. This is then processed by the liver and kidneys into active vitamin D, which supports healthy bones, immunity and overall vitality.

But our vitamin D-manufacturing capabilities evolved at a time when the human lifespan was considerably shorter and the consequences of cumulative UV exposure were perhaps less important. Our skin also makes vitamin D less efficiently as we age. And in the UK and other high-latitude countries, UVB rays are absent for much of the year. Even when they are present, the amount needed to generate sufficient vitamin D for our bodily needs varies enormously depending on skin tone and age. This makes it impossible to give universal advice on safe UVB exposure to get adequate vitamin D without risking either deficiency or skin damage.

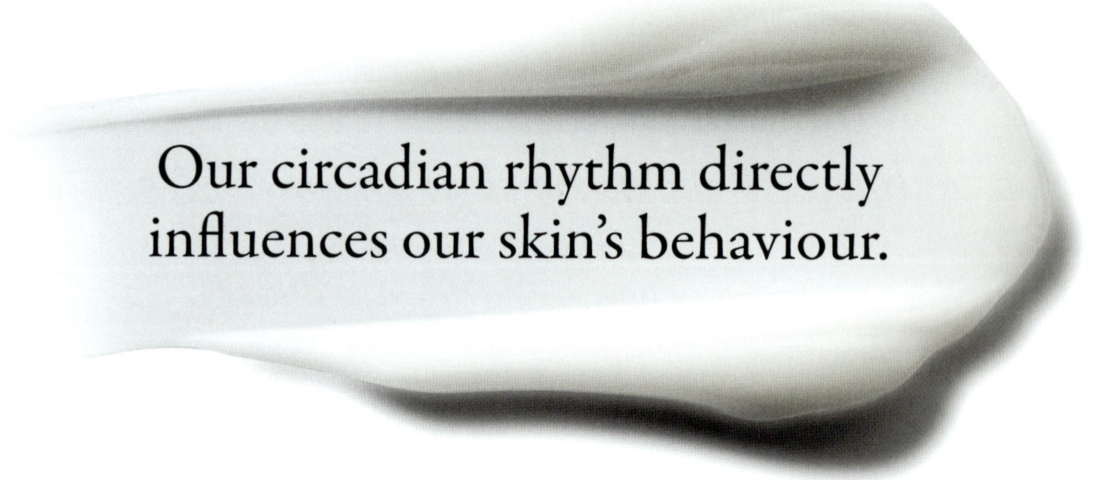

For these reasons, I recommend to patients that they take a daily vitamin D supplement; this ensures adequate levels of this important vitamin all year round for health, without needing to intentionally expose skin to harm.

THE INFLUENCE OF OUR CIRCADIAN RHYTHM

Exposure to natural light at the beginning and end of the day anchors our circadian rhythm, the body's internal 24-hour biological clock [i]. It tells you when to feel sleepy and when to feel awake, and it helps regulate hormones, digestion and overall wellbeing. A little low-level UVA also stimulates the release of nitric oxide, which supports vascular health and reduces cardiovascular risk.

Our circadian rhythm directly influences our skin's behaviour. It orchestrates activity across every skin cell, informing when our skin protects, repairs, regenerates and rests. Understanding this rhythm allows us to work with the schedule, rather than against it.

In the morning, our skin shifts into defence mode, strengthening its barrier function and increasing sebum production. Keratinocytes reinforce the skin barrier, locking in moisture and holding the line against incoming damage.

But as the evening approaches, our skin switches from defence to repair under the influence of melatonin. The barrier loosens slightly, making the skin more permeable. Cell division in the epidermis accelerates, DNA repair ramps up and blood flow to the skin increases. This makes evening the ideal time for applying active ingredients. Your skin is primed to absorb them and put them to work.

However, our circadian rhythm is easily disrupted. Whether it's thrown off by stress, jet-lag or a teething infant, barrier function can weaken, repair stalls and inflammation fires up. That's why quality sleep is so fundamental for healthy skin.

The bottom line:
In short, enjoy the light for your body clock and cardiovascular health, but protect your skin and let a supplement take care of your vitamin D.

THE SUN AND OXIDATIVE STRESS

We introduced reactive oxygen species (ROS) earlier (see page 29), when we looked at how UVA triggers immediate pigment darkening. However, the damage ROS cause extends far beyond pigmentation.

The first rule of thermodynamics is that energy cannot be created or destroyed; it can only be transformed. So, when sunlight hits the skin and isn't absorbed by melanin, that energy has to go somewhere. Other molecules in the skin, such as DNA, proteins and lipids, end up absorbing it instead.

One or two ROS may be neutralized harmlessly. But when enough are generated, they ignite a chain reaction that spreads through the cell, damaging everything in its path. The skin has its own network of antioxidant enzymes and molecules that work to neutralize ROS. But when the rate of production outpaces the rate of defence, the balance tips. This tipping point is called oxidative stress. Think of it as internal rust: slow, cumulative and largely invisible until the damage shows on the surface. Over time, it accelerates skin ageing and fuels the development of skin cancer.

UV isn't the only trigger. When inflammation becomes chronic rather than acute, it too generates ROS, adding to the oxidative burden. And crucially, oxidative stress and chronic inflammation are not just related – each drives the other. Oxidative stress triggers inflammatory pathways, and chronic inflammation generates more ROS. This self-reinforcing cycle is one of the central mechanisms of skin ageing.

WHAT IS OXIDATIVE STRESS?

Oxidative stress occurs when reactive oxygen species (ROS) overwhelm the skin's natural antioxidant defences.

Where do ROS come from?

External: UV light, pollution, cigarettes, alcohol, ultra-processed foods, and sugar.
Internal: Our mitochondria during normal cell metabolism, and chronic inflammation which, left unchecked, can become self-sustaining.

What do they do?

- ROS steal electrons from nearby molecules, damaging vital structures.
- DNA damage leads to mutations and increases skin cancer risk.
- Protein damage causes collagen and elastin breakdown, leading to wrinkles and sagging.
- Lipid damage weakens cell membranes and the skin barrier.
- Pigment pathway disruption leads to uneven skin tone.

Why it matters:

This invisible molecular damage is the central driver of skin ageing.

ESSENTIAL INFRASTRUCTURE

Your skin is far more than a simple covering. It is the body's largest organ, performing many vital functions.

It is responsive and intelligent, and its health closely reflects that of your entire body. It repairs, regenerates and protects with remarkable skill. Armed with this understanding of how your skin's structure and behaviour shape its needs, you now hold the keys to support it at every level.

Next, you'll learn how to work with your skin, using the most effective tools that science has to offer. This is where your skincare strategy truly begins.

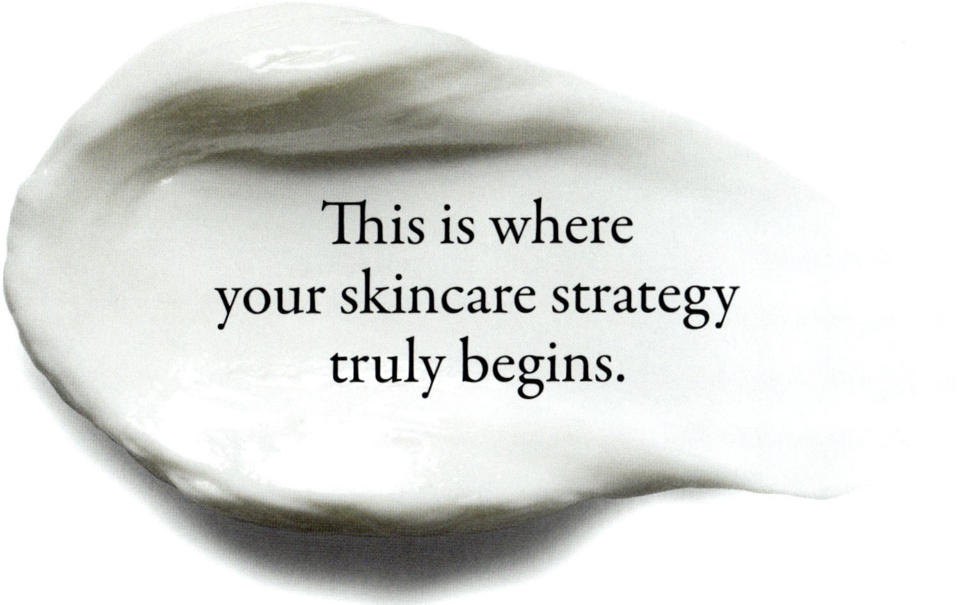

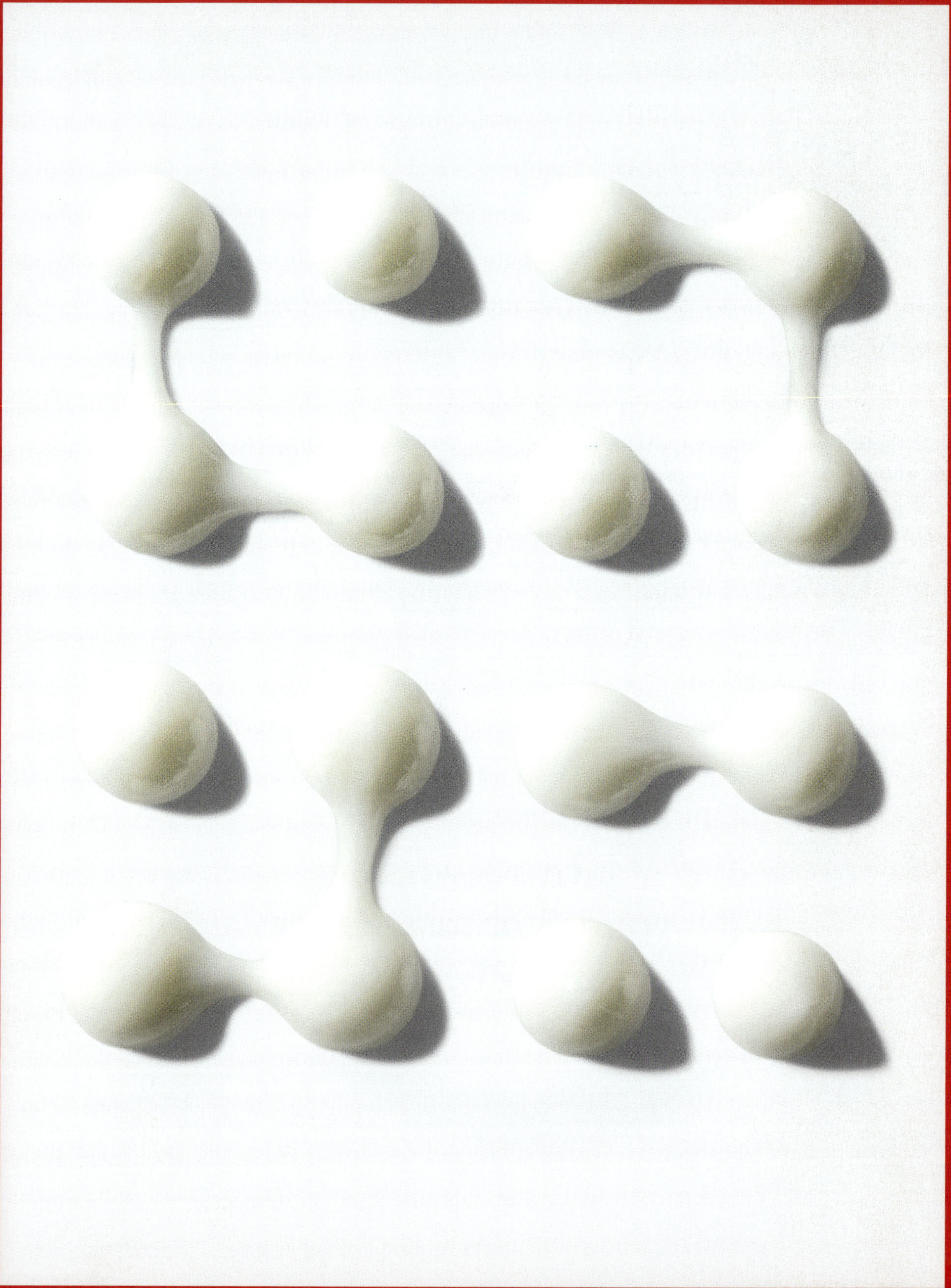

3

The Skin Type Preoccupation – Why Your Concern Matters More Than Your Type

THE ORIGINS OF SKIN TYPING

Walk up to any department-store beauty counter and one of the first questions you'll hear is: 'What's your skin type?'

It sounds intuitive. Scientific, even. But in my experience, it's neither. Since I began my practice, I've taken what some might call an audacious stance: I believe skin type doesn't matter nearly as much as we've been led to believe. In fact, it's a rather reductive lens that risks oversimplifying how skin actually behaves. To understand why skin typing still dominates, we need to trace it back to where it all began.

In the early 20th century, beauty pioneer Helena Rubinstein was perhaps the first entrepreneur to recognize the value of personalization in beauty. She had studied skin closely and observed that it behaved differently based on sebum production, which in turn influenced moisture retention. On this basis, she proposed three skin types: oily, combination and dry. This allowed her to recommend products tailored to her customers' individual needs and, perhaps more importantly, created an extremely effective marketing strategy that gave her an edge over her competitors. At this time the beauty world was limited to basic skin hygiene products or fragranced indulgences. Sunscreen wasn't invented until 1932 and we were not yet in the era of active ingredients.

Later on, the categories of normal and sensitive skin were added, when dermatologists in the 1970s and 1980s started paying attention to their patients' beauty habits, not just their diseases. Skin typing was subsequently adopted by legacy brands such as Clinique and Estée Lauder, becoming the gospel that shapes skincare marketing to this day.

THE 5 CLASSIC SKIN TYPES

Normal: Balanced.

Oily: Excessive sebum, shine, large pores.

Dry: Lacks moisture, rough, flaky, tight with invisible pores.

Sensitive: Reactive, prone to redness, itching or stinging.

Combination: Oily T-zone (forehead, nose, chin) with normal or dry cheeks.

THE MYTH OF 'NORMAL' SKIN

Here's a reality check: around 65 per cent of us have combination skin. That means combination skin is actually more . . . well . . . normal, than 'normal skin'.

The reason I focus on this is because it's the most common skin type, but also because it presents a challenge. How do you care for oily and dry skin simultaneously?

Something else worth noting: nearly 70 per cent of people now describe their skin as sensitive. That's the majority of us. It means many of us experience sensations such as itching, stinging or burning from time to time, along with visible signs such as redness, flaking or bumps. These reactions often have little to do with traditional skin types. Paradoxically, traditional skincare based on your skin type might actually be creating your sensitivity! It's a clear sign that the old-school labels we grew up with don't quite cut it anymore.

Combination or oily skin? Apply a single-ply tissue to your face upon waking. If the tissue is transparent only in the T-zone, you have combination skin. If it's transparent all over, your skin is oily.

THE FLAWLESS APPROACH:
FROM TYPE TO CONCERN

Instead of skin typing, I start with the concern right in front of me. From there, I reach into my toolkit of proven ingredients and pick the ones that fit. I support them with barrier-friendly basics, and treat *everyone* as if their skin is sensitive. After all, no one's ever been harmed by skincare formulated with sensitivity in mind.

This approach delivers better results and gives you a clear roadmap. It puts you back in control, helping you master your skin, instead of letting it master you.

THE BIG SIX SKIN CONCERNS

This is a list of the six most common concerns I see in the clinic and in my community online.

We'll get into the details of building a routine in the chapters to come. For now, let's focus on recognizing the Big Six skin concerns you're likely to face, regardless of skin type. This list isn't exhaustive, but I believe it captures enough of us to make this book worthwhile.

1 **Breakouts and Acne** (see opposite)

2 **Rosacea and Redness** (see page 52)

3 **Perioral Dermatitis (POD)** (see page 55)

4 **Pigmentation** (see page 57)

5 **Premature Ageing** (see page 62)

6 **Facial Eczema** (see page 65)

1 BREAKOUTS AND ACNE

Acne is the number one concern I treat in my Harley Street clinic. At least 80 per cent of my patients are women with acne, many in their thirties and beyond. When they arrive for the first time, they're looking for solutions across the full spectrum – from blemishes and blocked pores to pigmentation from previous spots and scarring. Many have suffered for decades, and the state of their skin colours everything they do.

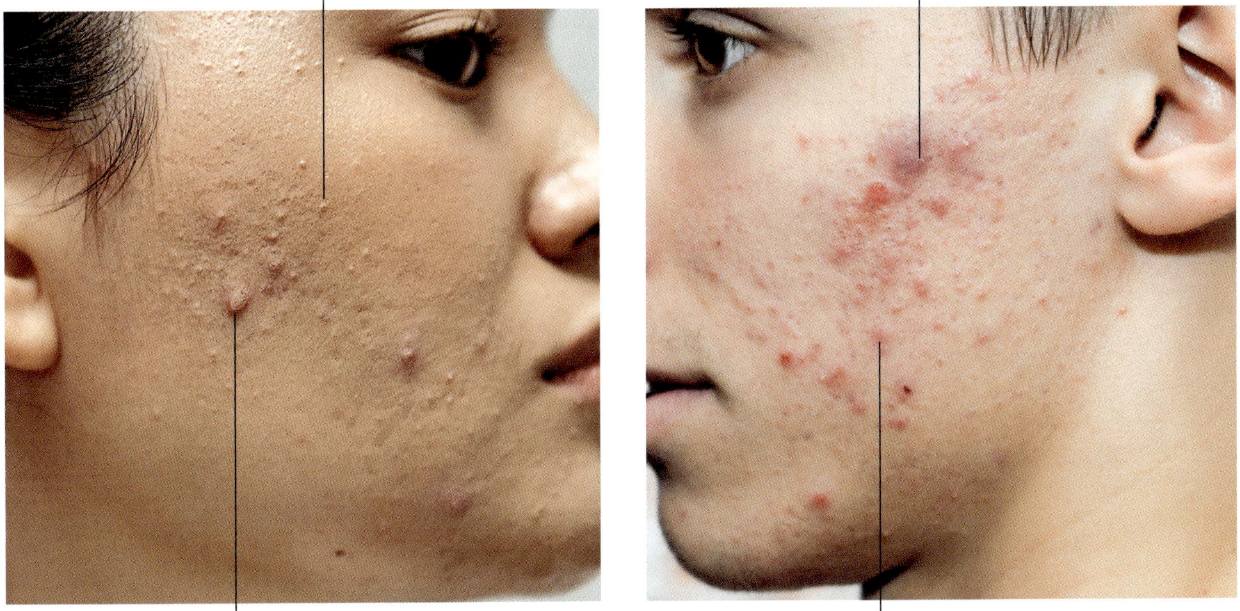

DIFFERENT PRESENTATIONS OF ACNE

WHAT EXACTLY IS ACNE?

Acne begins with trapped oil and dead skin cells blocking pores, creating comedones (see page 47). These can be open (exposed to air, visibly black due to oxidation) or closed (sealed off, appearing as small skin-coloured bumps that disturb the skin's texture, often only visible under harsh side-lighting). Over time, comedones can evolve into more obvious blemishes: small red spots known as papules, white-headed pustules and, in more severe cases, tender nodules or cysts lying deeper within the skin.

WHY DOES IT HAPPEN?

Things typically kick off with the hormones of puberty. Open comedones and a sheen of oil in the T-zone are usually the first signs, and the condition may spread to the upper back and chest, where freshly activated sebaceous glands cluster densely.

Interestingly, some populations, such as the hunter-gatherer Kitavan tribe in Papua New Guinea and the Aché people of Paraguay, escape acne almost entirely. Their genetics and diet, rich in fresh produce but low in refined sugar and dairy, are thought to be instrumental.

WHOM DOES IT AFFECT THE MOST?

Teens are the hardest hit – up to 80 per cent will be affected in the Western world (especially around exam time).[ii] But it doesn't stop there: around 40 per cent of adult women also struggle with persistent or late-onset acne at some point.[iii] Hormonal shifts, whether due to contraception changes, pregnancy, IVF, menopause, or even the menstrual cycle (premenstrual breakouts affect 70 per cent of women) are common triggers. Mix in stress or the wrong skincare for extra provocation. Men get adult acne too, but women are affected up to twice as often.

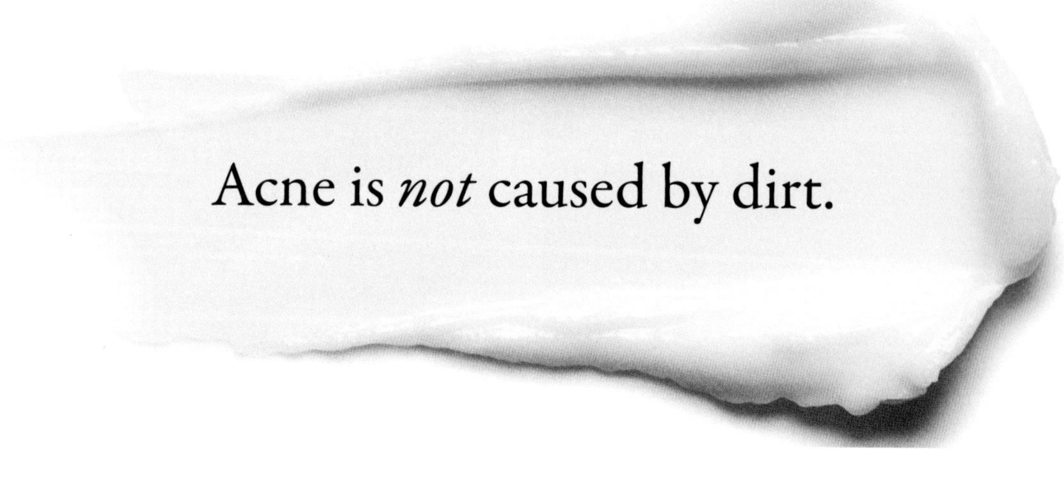

COMMON ACNE MYTHS:
CLEARING UP THE CONFUSION

1

You're not clean enough

Acne isn't the result of being dirty. Overcleansing is actually counterproductive, stripping your skin barrier and cranking up inflammation.

2

You'll grow out of it

Many don't. Some have clear skin by their twenties, when their hormones settle down after puberty, but often a long-term approach to continuously treat and prevent breakouts is necessary. The upside? Many acne-fighting ingredients are also gold standard for tackling premature ageing.

3

You can spot-treat your way out of acne

Acne is a whole-skin condition. Spot-by-spot reactivity is unlikely to solve the problem, because multiple pores get blocked simultaneously within the acne-prone zones. Unplugging them all at once is core to stabilizing your skin.

4

Sun exposure helps

Tanning is never a solution. UVB rays (that burn the skin) offer temporary anti-inflammatory relief that can lessen the red, swollen nature of breakouts. But they can also trigger more congested pores and darken existing pigmentation marks from old spots. This means that when you stop tanning, things often look much worse. Then, of course, there's the premature ageing aspect of UV exposure to consider...

5

Make-up causes acne

It can – but it doesn't have to. Longwear foundation, for instance, can be highly occlusive to pores and near-impossible to remove, often requiring double cleansing with oils or balms – products that are potentially disastrous for acne-prone skin. (See page 51 for make-up advice.)

6

There's something wrong with your hormones

In adult women, breakouts tend to shift away from the T-zone to the U of the face, along the chin and jawline. It's frequently labelled 'hormonal acne', however I'd argue that all female acne is inherently hormonal in nature.

For the majority of adult female acne sufferers, cycles are regular and hormones reassuringly normal. I don't have a good explanation for why the pattern of acne changes in women. There seems to be a shift in the sensitivity of androgen receptors in the oil glands along the jawline, rather than changes in hormone levels themselves.

7 'It's just a few spots'

I've lost count of the instances when patients have told me how the casual dismissal of their skin issues has crushed their spirit. Everyone sees their skin through their own unique lens of experience. I've seen utter indifference from someone with widespread, scarring acne. I've witnessed acute anguish from someone with prominent pores and occasional blemishes. Both deserve help, as skin issues can have a tremendous impact on our mental state and wellbeing.

8 Treatments work by drying out your skin

It's easy to think that acne treatments are working by sucking the oil out of your skin, because it feels dry and flaky, and that somehow this *needs* to happen for them to be effective. That's not the case. In reality, dryness is a side effect, not the mechanism through which the treatment is working. It can be completely avoided and should be, as it might aggravate existing blemishes. Treat acne-prone skin as though it's inherently sensitive from the start by supporting your skin barrier with the right products (see pages 117 and 138), and your results will be far better. Most acne patients need more moisturizer than they think.

9 You can eat your way to a solution

I've looked after many nutritionists with impeccable diets suffering from acne over the years. A balanced diet is part of a holistic acne management plan, but it's unlikely to solve things alone. Acne is mostly influenced by genetics and hormones. That said, what you eat can tip the scales. High-glycaemic foods – sugary drinks, white bread, pastries, ultra-processed snacks – can worsen breakouts by driving up blood sugar and insulin levels, which in turn nudge oil glands into overdrive and fuel inflammation. Dairy, especially skimmed milk, can have similar effects in those who are already acne-prone. I favour moderation. Don't obsess over cutting things out, but if dairy worsens your skin, stick to one good whole milk flat white a day rather than five skinny lattes. Focus on eating for calm skin: plenty of colourful vegetables, healthy fats from oily fish and nuts, and low-glycaemic carbs, such as sweet potatoes and brown rice.

HOW TO IDENTIFY ACNE

Comedones: Closed (skin-coloured bumps) or open (blackheads).

Red bumps: Papules, pustules or nodules or cysts, clustered in typical acne zones (see page 48).

Pattern: Distribution across face, chest and back (unlike other skin conditions).

Aftermath: Flat red/brown marks (known as post-inflammatory hyperpigmentation/PIH) or indented scars from deeper lesions.

Key distinction: Comedones present (unlike rosacea or periorificial dermatitis).

MAKE-UP AND ACNE

It's natural to want to apply make-up to cover up acne, but it can be a vicious cycle: you reach for cosmetics that promise not to budge but, unfortunately, many of these formulas are inherently pore-blocking and extremely stubborn to remove, leading to a downward spiral. Skin gets more congested and irritated, increasing the desire to conceal... and things go from bad to worse.

My philosophy on this is to skip anything that adds longevity to make-up, such as setting sprays or powders. For oil control, stick to the simple practice of using blotting papers. Also, avoid anything that is meant to cover skin for an extended period of time, such as longwear foundation (why anyone needs 24-hour coverage, I have no clue). Choose cosmetics labelled non-comedogenic (meaning they're unlikely to block your pores) and focus coverage *only where it's needed* using a highly pigmented concealer that allows for pinpoint application. Use a tiny paintbrush to apply it, then use a finger to roll the edges of the concealer to blend. This avoids unnecessary coverage where it's not needed, so skin still looks like skin.

Make-up maestro Isamaya Ffrench has a tutorial on YouTube demonstrating her 'crosshatch' concealer technique which I often share with my patients. As a base, use a light foundation/tinted moisturizer/tinted sunscreen to even out the skin's appearance, then reapply concealer as needed on the go with a small brush and clean fingers.

2 ROSACEA AND REDNESS

Rosacea is so similar to acne in its presentation that it was actually called 'acne rosacea' until recently, although they're unrelated disorders.

Around 5 per cent of the world's population suffers from some form of rosacea.[iv] We're often reluctant to discuss it because prolonged blushing has emotional connotations, such as embarrassment or shame. That feeling can itself promote the blush. Fortunately, growing openness around skin health, particularly on social media, is beginning to dismantle that stigma.

WHAT EXACTLY IS ROSACEA?

Rosacea is a mixture of things. First, we might see excitable blood vessels that widen too much with very little provocation, as the blood flows very close to the skin's surface, creating a flush. It might happen when you pop indoors after being out in the cold, or when you sip on a mug of hot tea. Harmless, but annoying.

Next, there's an overexuberant immune system. It's there to protect us against the environment, but it's a bit trigger-happy, getting hot and bothered by skincare that's drying or acidic

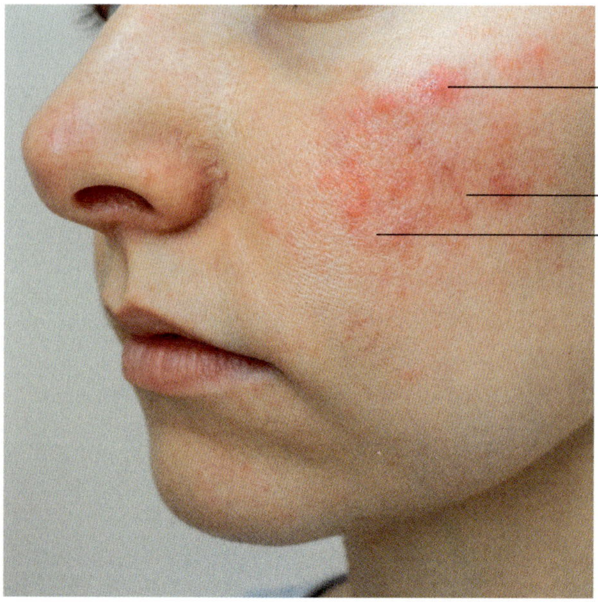

ROSACEA

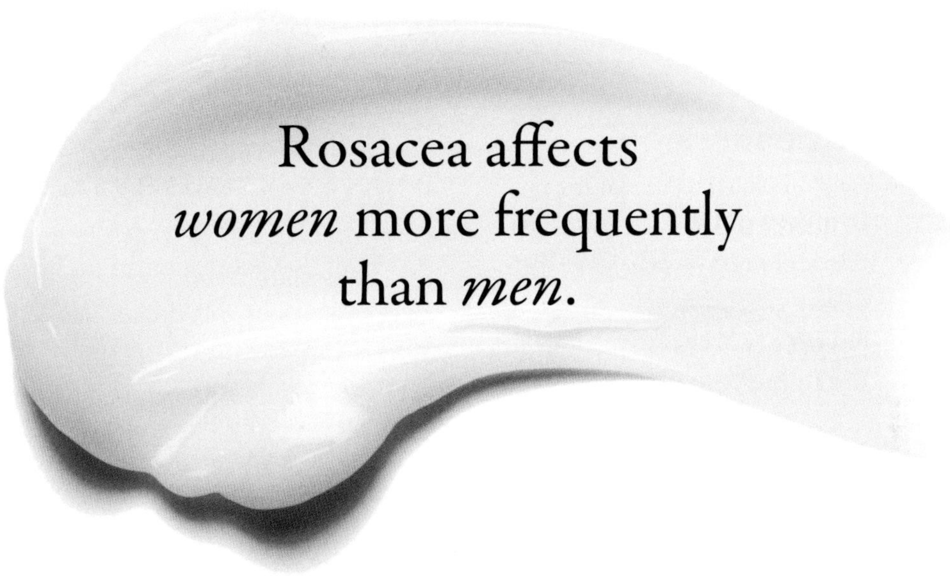

Rosacea affects *women* more frequently than *men*.

(such as a serum containing vitamin C). I liken it to a fire alarm going off when the kettle boils, rather than if the oven is ablaze. An unhappy skin barrier also features – most people will describe their skin as 'sensitive'.

Finally, acne-like changes can appear – we see those red papules and pustules again. But here's what's critical: no comedones. Background redness sits in the middle of the face, over the curvy surface of the cheeks and chin rather than the typical T-zone or jawline we see with acne. The spots themselves are more mound-like, rather than pointed. Hills not mountains, if you will.

WHY DOES IT HAPPEN?

The rosacea story is a multifaceted one. Genetics are definitely a key player, as it's much more common in certain parts of the world, such as Northern Europe, in people with light eyes and white skin. If your parents were flushed after a glass of red wine, chances are you might be too. Beyond that, it's a tussle between your innate immune system and the nerve endings that plug into the blood vessels. The microbiome is probably not a passive bystander either – it's likely that both the gut and skin microbiome are implicated. Basically, it's complicated.

WHOM DOES IT AFFECT THE MOST?

Rosacea typically kicks in after the age of 30, affecting women more frequently than men, although men may experience more severe disease, with thickening of the skin due to fibrosis, often over the nose. This is known as phymatous change.

COMMON ROSACEA MYTHS:
CLEARING UP THE CONFUSION

1 Drinkers get it

Alcohol aggravates rosacea by dilating blood vessels, especially red wine (which also releases histamine). But it's not the cause.

2 Facials are a good idea

No, definitely not. Neither are beauty boxes or bundles. Or using your friend's products. Your skin needs rigorous simplicity and zero deviation from a carefully planned minimalist routine. Rosacea doesn't like surprises.

3 Rosacea only affects the skin

This often surprises people. The eyes are frequently affected (in around 40 per cent of sufferers), so if you're rubbing gritty eyes with poor tear film (the coating on the surface of your eye), it might be ocular rosacea. It can also present in the eyes first, so your optometrist may be the person who makes the diagnosis.

HOW TO IDENTIFY ROSACEA

- **Persistent redness** in the centre of the face with broken capillaries.
- **Flushing** (prolonged blushing).
- **Papules and pustules** that are red and round-topped (more mound-like than acne's pointed blemishes).
- **Stinging or burning** from skincare products.
- **No comedones** (blocked pores).
- **Eyes** that feel gritty or dry.
- **Unaffected nasolabial folds** (nose-to-mouth creases).
- **Phymatous change** (skin thickening).

3 PERIORAL DERMATITIS (POD)

POD is skin inflammation around the mouth. It's a bit of a fiend as we don't understand it well and it often masquerades as other conditions such as rosacea, acne or seborrhoeic dermatitis. Misdiagnosis as the latter can lead to unnecessary topical steroid use and dramatic rebound when withdrawn, so getting the diagnosis right is crucial.

WHAT EXACTLY IS POD?

POD has a very characteristic appearance – lots of tiny red bumps that all look alike (unlike the varied blemishes of acne and rosacea) – clustering around the mouth but characteristically sparing the skin directly next to the lip edge. The surface may be dry and flaky. It can also appear around the eyes (periocular dermatitis) and, if severe, spread onto the upper cheeks.

WHY DOES IT HAPPEN?

No one really knows what causes this problem, but fussy skincare routines are often involved, along with the use of topical steroids (especially the stronger forms). Other triggers can include fluoridated toothpaste and nasal steroid inhalers.

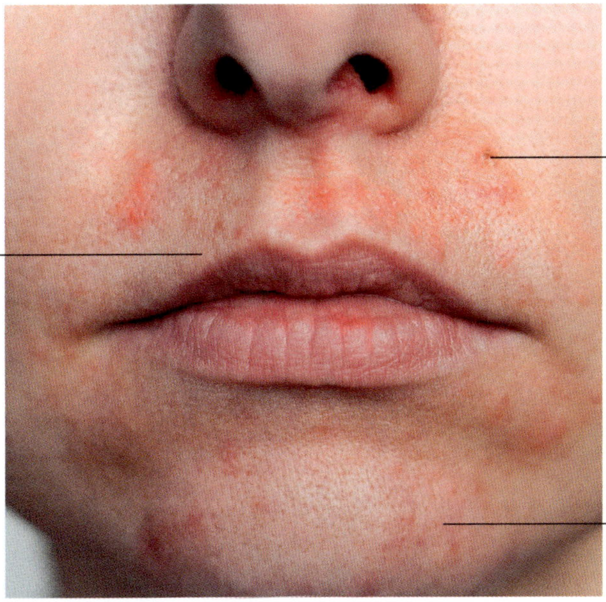

PERIORAL DERMATITIS

It's also set off by stress, in common with most other inflammatory skin issues. There's often an episode of skin-barrier upset in the early stages, which perhaps then leads to the penetration of chemicals in our personal care products that aren't meant to get in. This drives inflammation, the barrier becomes more damaged and a vicious cycle is created where every product starts to sting or burn.

WHOM DOES IT AFFECT THE MOST?

It mostly affects women – only about 10 per cent of sufferers are men.

HOW TO IDENTIFY POD

- History of steroid use
- No comedones
- No flushing
- Mouth-to-nose rash sparing the lip edge

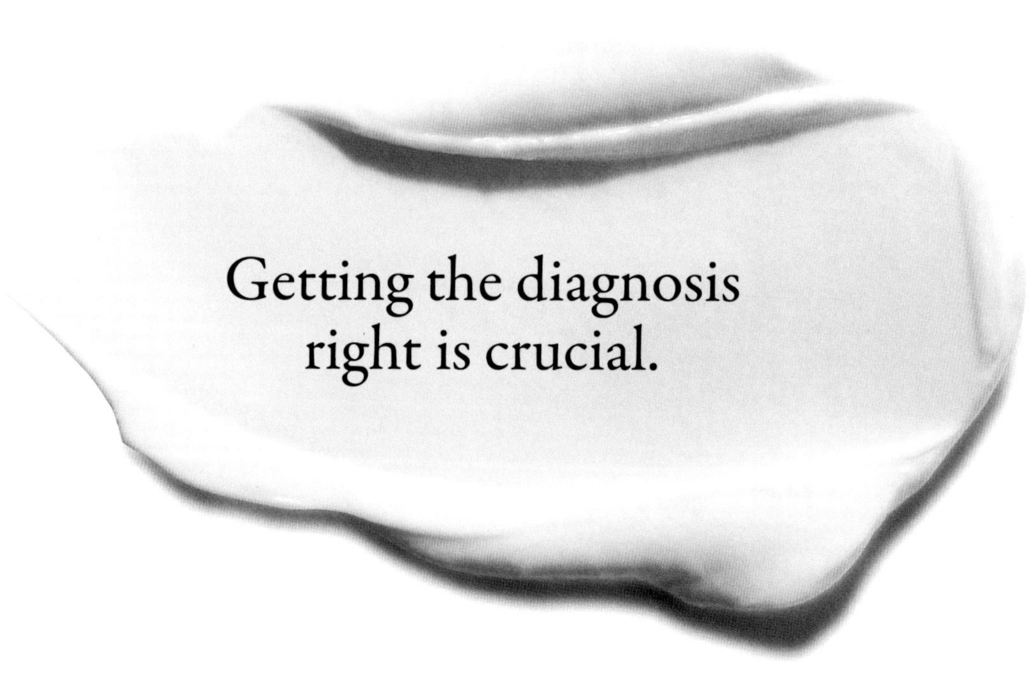

4 PIGMENTATION

Pigmentation is the umbrella term for conditions that are caused by excess melanin in the skin (see pages 28–9). It's wonderful to treat, as a smart skincare routine can often make a tremendous impact in a short timeframe.

When the pigment system misfires, too much melanin gets deposited in patches, leading to uneven skin tone. Because our brains instinctively associate uniform skin with health, these changes are often a source of cosmetic frustration even when skin otherwise functions well.

A word on terminology. You might be wondering: is it pigmentation or hyperpigmentation? Basically, they mean the same thing. The prefix 'hyper' in medicine just means 'a lot', so I use pigmentation for the sake of brevity.

THE TOP THREE TYPES

Here are the top three causes of pigmentation and uneven skin tone I see in the clinic.

1

Solar lentigines (also known as sun spots or age spots)
Flat, round, brown marks on sun-exposed areas, such as the temples, forehead and cheekbones. Larger and more permanent than freckles, they don't change much in appearance with the season.

2

Post-acne marks
Red or brown footprints left behind after breakouts heal, or when a blemish gets picked or squeezed. They align with your acne pattern and can cause just as much distress as the blemishes themselves. They are often mistakenly called 'scars', but post-acne marks are pigmentation, not structural skin damage. This is an important distinction, as it makes them significantly more treatable.

3

Melasma
Distinctive, symmetrical, map-like patches of grey or brown pigmentation that are seen on the forehead, the cheekbones and the upper lip.

WHY DOES IT HAPPEN?

The sun's UV rays are a major driving force for pigmentation, which shouldn't come as a surprise given melanin's protective role as the skin's neighbourhood watch. Solar lentigines result from cumulative UV rays over decades. Over time, the melanocytes in our skin become tired and jaded; they've seen it all and now they respond almost automatically, by sounding the alarm and producing melanin in the same spots.

UV isn't the only culprit – recent studies tell us that pollution also has a role to play in triggering our skin's defences. Tiny particles of soot in the air from road traffic and industry can actually penetrate the skin barrier and set off the alarm system too. The melanocytes get stimulated, driving them to overproduce melanin.

In post-acne marks, the neighbourhood watch is responding to an actual disturbance in the skin – an inflamed blemish. As we saw in Chapter 2 (see pages 23–41), once the trouble is dealt with, the watch stays wary and on patrol, producing melanin even though the threat has passed.

On the other hand, melasma is caused by hyper-excitable melanocytes in zones of the face that are unusually sensitive to oestrogen and progestogen. When exposed to provoking factors such as UV, they tend to spill excess melanin into the skin.

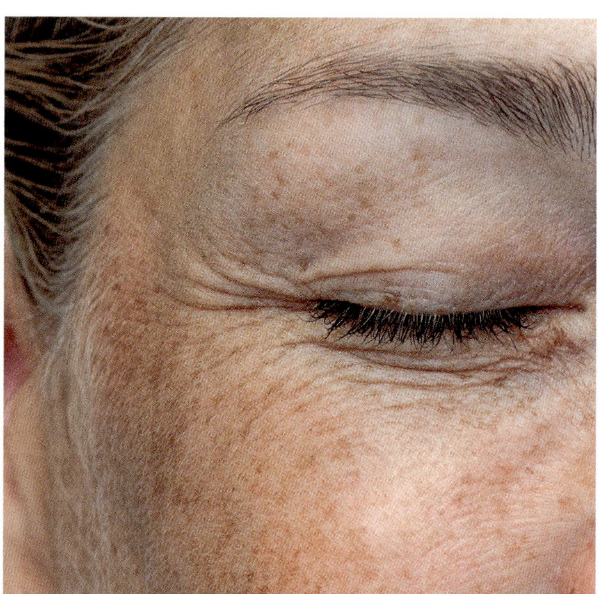

SOLAR LENTIGINES

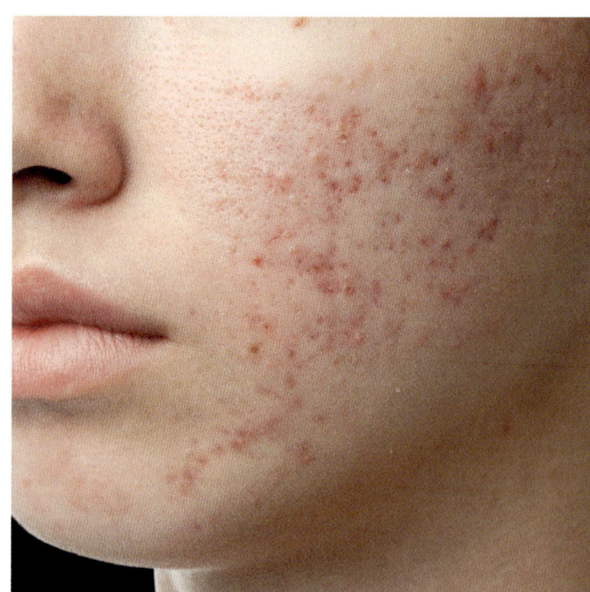

POST-ACNE MARKS

They behave a bit like an overzealous neighbour, always at the curtain, looking for danger and sending up lots of false alarms. They also have memory, meaning that even if you manage to clear up the pigment from one episode, getting caught off guard again without sunscreen even for a few minutes can send you back to square one.

WHOM DOES IT AFFECT THE MOST?

White-skinned individuals over the age of 50 are at risk of solar lentigines, especially with high lifetime UV exposure. Almost everyone with acne gets marks left behind when their blemish disappears, but those with more ferocious inflammation or those with darker skin will fuel more persistent pigment.

Melasma – sometimes called the 'mask of pregnancy' – has strong hormonal associations. Up to a quarter of affected women experience it during pregnancy or after starting hormonal contraception. As a result, only about 10 per cent of those with melasma are men. Genetics are strongly implicated, as is exposure to both UV and visible light. Melasma is not only one of the most stubborn forms of pigmentation, it's also the most misunderstood. I've seen countless patients who've been given confusing, even harmful advice. Over the page I'll tackle some of the most common myths I hear about melasma and replace them with the facts.

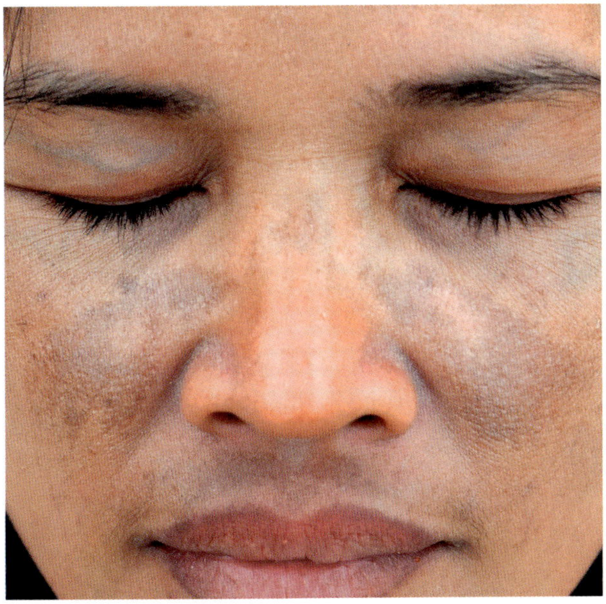

MELASMA

HOW TO IDENTIFY PIGMENTATION

Solar lentigines: Small, well-defined brown spots scattered unevenly across sun-exposed areas.

Post-acne marks: Flat marks sitting exactly where spots healed, irregular shapes, no symmetry.

Melasma: Larger, soft-edged patches, typically symmetrical in a map-like pattern.

COMMON MELASMA MYTHS:
CLEARING UP THE CONFUSION

1

I don't need to wear sunscreen indoors

It's true that the level of risk indoors varies. If you're sitting well away from windows, in a shaded room, your exposure to UV is very low. But if you're close to a window, particularly with strong daylight streaming through (think of a sunny morning at your desk or a long drive in the car), UVA rays can still reach your skin through glass. The risk also depends on the time of year, your latitude, and how much shade is outside the window from things like trees and buildings.

The problem is, all of this is tricky to calculate in real life. In my experience, the simplest and most effective approach is to make sunscreen a non-negotiable part of your morning routine. Apply it every day, regardless of the weather, and reapply if you'll be spending time outdoors. This takes the guesswork out of sun protection – rather than trying to judge the conditions, you're consistently covered.

While not all indoor light exposure is equally risky, building the habit of daily sunscreen use removes the guesswork and offers the best protection against melasma recurrence.

2

I need to scrub away pigmentation

Definitely not. This brings to mind a case I saw for a TV show I presented back in 2015 (TLC's *Extreme Beauty Disasters*). A woman who wanted help for her pigmentation came on for advice and treatment. She had been having microdermabrasion, a procedure that involves using physical exfoliation, often by spraying skin with fine crystals to mechanically buff away the top layers of the skin. When the pigmentation wasn't showing signs of improvement, the therapist stepped it up and things got worse. When she came on the show, her melasma was in freefall.

Hypersensitive melanocytes don't like friction. While exfoliation can help eliminate excess melanin inside keratinocytes, using precise chemistry to dissolve bonds between dead cells – rather than brute force – is the way to go.

3

Once it's gone, it's gone

Alas, no. Melasma is chronic and relapsing, tending to linger for years or even decades, so it needs a maintenance strategy.

4

Hydroquinone is toxic

Hydroquinone remains the gold-standard treatment for pigmentation, including melasma. But it often attracts controversy around its safety. In truth, when prescribed appropriately by a physician, hydroquinone is both safe and very effective.

Most of the concern comes from misuse. In many parts of the world, so-called 'whitening creams' are sold without medical supervision, in unlicensed beauty salons. They often contain hydroquinone at concentrations that far exceed the standard 2–4 per cent used in dermatology. In these unregulated products, the risk of complications rises sharply, including exogenous ochronosis, a paradoxical condition where the skin becomes darker and more mottled instead of lighter. That's why context and supervision matter. With a proper diagnosis and correctly dosed prescription, hydroquinone can be used safely and strategically, often in a limited treatment course (no longer than three months at a time) and in rotation with other pigmentation solutions.

5 Blue light from screens is the problem

This light is a fraction of the intensity of that coming from the sun. Studies suggest screens don't contribute to melasma.[v]

6 Lasers are the answer

This is one of the most common misconceptions about melasma, and one of the riskiest. I would categorically advise against starting treatment for melasma with lasers. There's a significant risk of making things worse, as laser energy can easily excite the same overactive melanocytes that drive melasma in the first place. While lasers can be considered later (but only in experienced hands), they're never a first-line treatment. If topical treatments fail, it's crucial to pre-treat the skin with a pigment suppressor such as hydroquinone to calm the overactive melanocytes before attempting any in-clinic intervention.

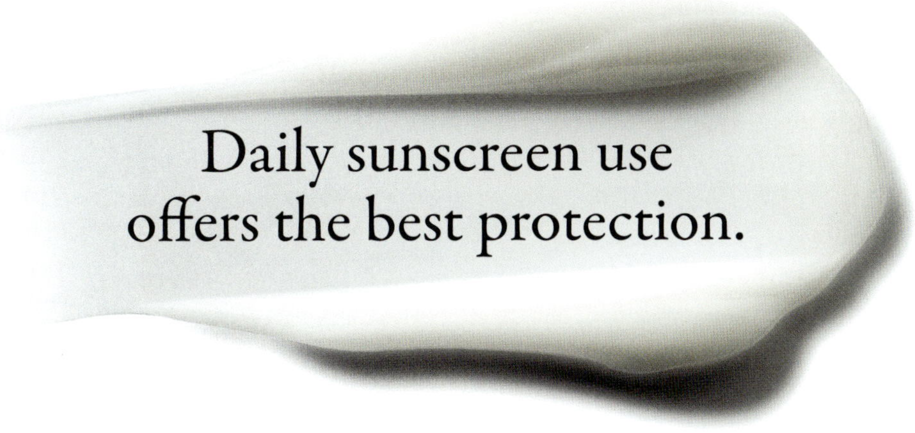

5 PREMATURE AGEING

Premature ageing means your skin starts to look older than your biological age, and it creeps up gradually. In the clinic, I often hear the complaint: 'I look tired even when I'm not.' Or there's a disconnect between what someone sees in the mirror versus how youthful and energetic they feel. The main culprit is cumulative UVA exposure and the many ways it insidiously alters how our skin looks and functions over time.

WHAT EXACTLY IS PREMATURE AGEING?

Premature ageing shows up as a myriad of signs etched into the skin: fine lines, deeper wrinkles, uneven skin tone, texture changes, loss of elasticity and sagging. It will also tend to look dull and sallow, and broken capillaries can appear. The skin barrier is impaired and skin may be more reactive. You'll typically notice wrinkles forming around your eyes, on your forehead and around your mouth first, as facial expressions leave their mark.

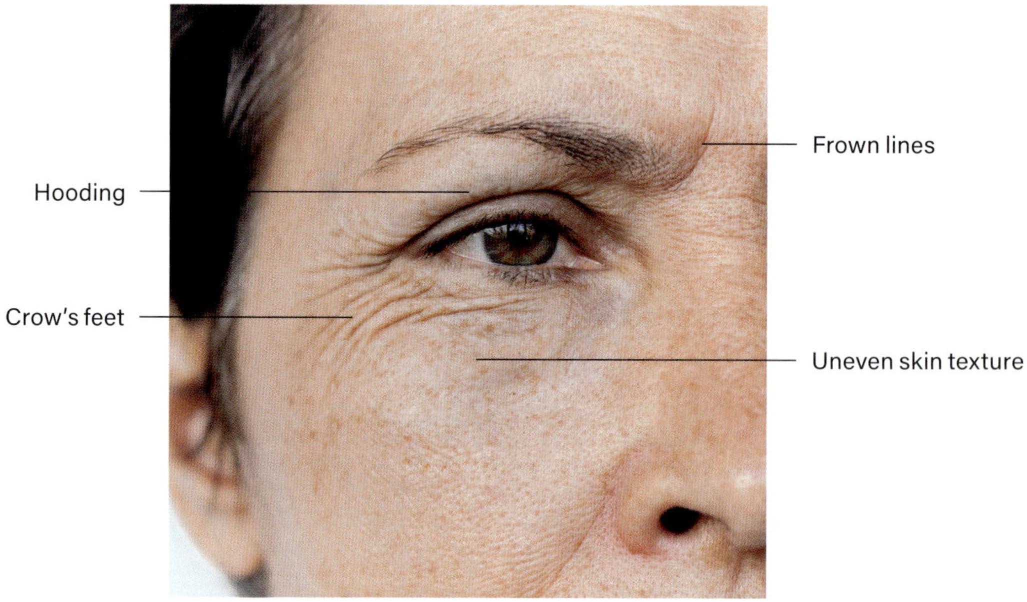

PREMATURE AGEING

While premature ageing tends to show up earlier and more visibly in lighter skin tones – especially through lines and sagging – those with deeper skin tones are not immune. It may manifest differently: as uneven texture, dullness or pigmentation rather than fine lines.

WHY DOES IT HAPPEN?

Inflammaging – a type of ageing that is due to chronic inflammation – is at the heart of premature skin ageing. Inflammation is meant to switch on speedily, deal with a problem, then switch off before it does harm to our own tissues. However, when it becomes chronic due to oxidative stress (see page 40), it rumbles on at low levels, breaking down collagen and elastin while creating more reactive oxygen species (see page 40) in a vicious cycle. Think of it like internal rust.

UV is the dominant force driving inflammaging in our skin, but smoking, pollution, stress and poor sleep are also co-conspirators.

Tightly connected to inflammaging is a process called glycation. This is where excess sugar from our diet interacts with collagen and elastin, causing it to become stiff, much like caramel hardening. These are called Advanced Glycation End-products (or AGEs – not difficult to remember!). Not only do they weaken the structure of the dermis, they also drive yet more inflammation.

WHOM DOES IT AFFECT THE MOST?

Those with lighter skin tones and frequent UV exposure are most susceptible. Think of a tan as an environmental tax – you'll pay for it later in lines and wrinkles. The tax is doubled for sunbed use – there is no safe way to use a tanning bed.

As we explored in Chapter 2, lifestyle compounds this further – the same triggers that drive oxidative stress accelerate inflammaging too. Smoking, pollution, Western diets with ultra-processed foods and high-glycaemic loads all contribute through their ability to drive oxidative stress, chronic inflammation and glycation.

COMMON PREMATURE AGEING MYTHS:
CLEARING UP THE CONFUSION

1

I don't need SPF unless it's sunny
UVA penetrates clouds, windows and windscreens, and it's present all year round. Even on gloomy winter days, your skin accumulates damage.

2

Anti-ageing products are snake oil
While there are admittedly many products on the market that overpromise and underdeliver, ingredients such as retinoids and antioxidants are backed by a wealth of solid scientific evidence and are proven to significantly slow down and improve signs of ageing, as we'll see in Chapter 5 (see pages 89–119).

3

I can't see the damage, so it's not happening
By the time fine lines or pigmentation appear, the underlying damage has been accumulating for years.

4

Only expensive products work
Many of the most proven ingredients, such as retinoids, niacinamide and SPF, are now available at accessible price points.

HOW TO IDENTIFY PREMATURE AGEING

- Lines that linger when you stop smiling or frowning
- Uneven skin texture or tone
- Brown spots and visible broken capillaries
- Dullness or sallowness
- Loss of bounce or firmness
- Sagging
- Slow healing time

6 FACIAL ECZEMA

If your face is red, dry and irritated, the temptation is to call it 'eczema' and reach for the hydrocortisone cream. But facial eczema is not one condition, it's several, and knowing which one you're dealing with matters because the triggers, the location on the body and how we deal with it are different. It's helpful to start by identifying the differences between the types of eczema first.

Atopic eczema favours the eyelids, the neck and the skin around the mouth. It's often part of a bigger picture: you may have had eczema as a child, or asthma or hay fever run in the family. Your skin is dry and itchy and tends to flare and settle in cycles, during which the skin looks red and feels rough, with fine scaling.

Seborrhoeic eczema looks quite different. It sits in the eyebrows, the nasal folds and the hairline – the areas where sebaceous glands are most active. It's often flaky with a slightly yellowish, greasy scale, and can overlap with dandruff on the scalp.

Irritant dermatitis is reactive. It shows up wherever something has aggravated the skin. Affected areas look red, feel raw and may sting, sometimes with surface scaling or even weeping. Common sites include around the eyes or on the cheeks.

Allergic contact dermatitis can mimic any of the forms above, but the clue is in the pattern: it often maps to wherever the allergen has been applied and persists or recurs until the culprit is identified and removed. The exception is thin-skinned areas such as the eyelids and neck, which can react to products applied elsewhere on the face or body, making them early warning sites. The affected area looks red and swollen, often with intense itch

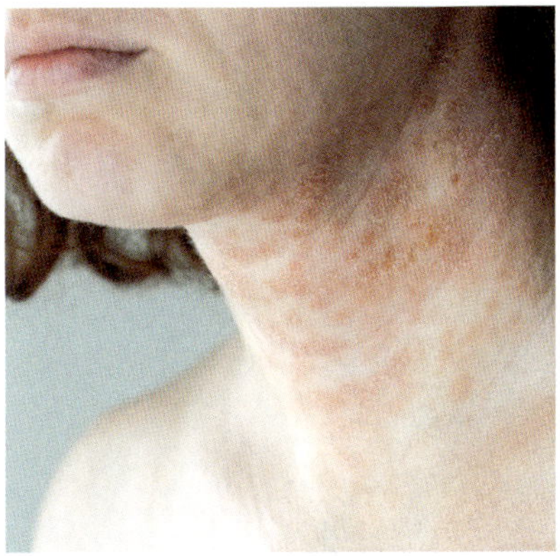

ATOPIC ECZEMA

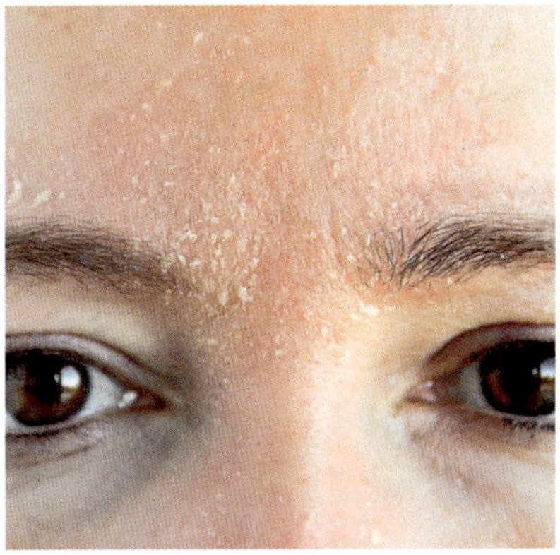

SEBORRHOEIC ECZEMA

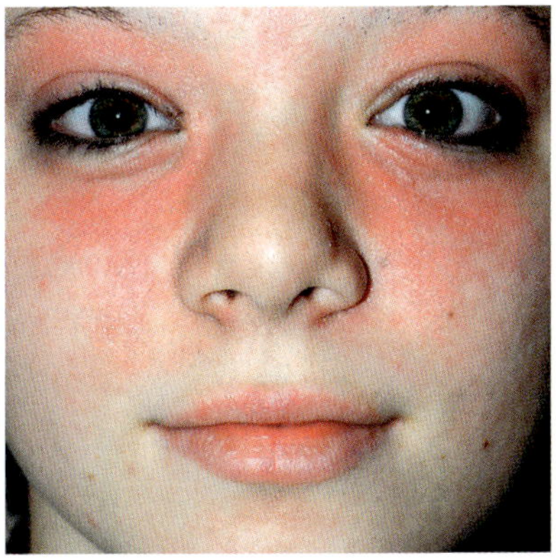

ALLERGIC CONTACT DERMATITIS

and occasionally small blisters. Common triggers include fragrances, preservatives and hair dye.

WHO DOES IT AFFECT THE MOST?

Women are most at risk of irritant and allergic contact dermatitis due to more frequent skincare use. Seborrhoeic eczema is more common in men, due to higher androgen activity. Atopic eczema is slightly more common in women.

COMMON ATOPIC ECZEMA MYTHS: CLEARING UP THE CONFUSION

1

It's contagious
This is one of the most damaging myths – and it's false. Eczema isn't caused by a virus or bacteria you can 'catch'. You cannot spread it through touch. The stigma this myth creates causes real psychological harm to sufferers who already feel self-conscious about their skin.

2

You'll grow out of it
While many children do see improvement as they age, atopic eczema can persist into adulthood or even appear for the first time in your thirties, forties or beyond. Adult-onset eczema is increasingly common.

3

It's just dry skin
Dry skin is a symptom of eczema, but eczema is a complex disorder involving barrier dysfunction, immune system overactivity and genetics. The inflammation, itching and susceptibility to infection go far beyond simple dryness.

4

Stress causes eczema
Stress doesn't cause eczema, but it's certainly a significant trigger for flare-ups. When stressed, our bodies release cortisol, which can disrupt our skin barrier and increase inflammation. Managing stress is important, but it won't prevent eczema in someone who is predisposed to it.

HOW TO IDENTIFY ECZEMA

Skin changes:
Scaling , flaking, redness, itching

Eyelids and neck:
Irritant, allergic or atopic eczema

Nasal folds and eyebrows:
Seborrhoeic eczema

5 Diet can cure eczema

I've looked after many patients experiencing eczema flares, despite eating all the right things. Your diet can support skin health but it isn't a treatment for eczema. True food allergies aside, restrictive elimination diets should only be pursued with proper guidance, as they can do more harm than good.

6 Natural products are better

Natural ingredients can be helpful (such as shea butter) and unhelpful (tea tree oil can irritate *and* cause allergies). Choose fragrance-free, minimalist formulas designed for compromised barriers – regardless of whether they're marketed as 'natural'.

7 It's due to poor hygiene

Au contraire. Being too clean is likely to be far more problematic, as overwashing disturbs your microbiome, expels helpful, water-retaining lipids and weakens your skin barrier.

8 You should avoid bathing

Just don't languish in hot baths loaded with essential oils. Lukewarm water, gentle cleansers and moisturizing immediately afterwards is the best approach.

9 Steroids are dangerous

This is a great example of how dose is everything. Topical steroids are helpful *when used correctly* – correct strength, right location, appropriate duration. The big worry is skin thinning, which is only seen with incorrect or excessive use. It's more common to see patients suffering needlessly because steroid phobia has prevented them from getting relief.

THE KEY TAKEAWAY

Location, distribution and **history** will get you most of the way when it comes to figuring out which type of eczema you're dealing with. If the condition is symmetrical and longstanding, think atopic. If it follows the oily zones, think seborrhoeic. If it appeared after a change in routine, think irritant. And if the eczema keeps coming back in the same spot despite everything you've tried, consider contact allergy and get patch tested by a dermatologist.

WHEN TO SEE A DERMATOLOGIST

A good skincare routine can achieve a lot, but there are times when your skin needs more than over-the-counter products can offer. Here's when I'd recommend booking an appointment.

Urgent

- Any mole that has changed in size, shape, colour or texture, or that bleeds, itches or crusts. Don't delay on this.
- Acne that is scarring, painful or not responding to over-the-counter treatments. Early intervention prevents permanent damage.
- A flare of eczema or rosacea that is escalating despite your usual routine.
- A new rash that isn't getting better after two weeks.
- Skin that has become suddenly and persistently reactive without any obvious cause.

Worth a consultation

- Pigmentation that is worsening, spreading or not responding to topical treatment after three months.
- Persistent dark circles. Hollowing, sagging or loss of facial fullness that skincare can't address.
- Any skin concern that is affecting your confidence or quality of life. That alone is reason enough.
- While care of the scalp is beyond the scope of this book, if you're experiencing hair thinning or hair loss, a dermatologist can help.

What to expect

A good dermatologist will take a full history, examine your skin and, if needed, arrange further investigations. They should also review your current routine. Don't be embarrassed to bring your products along. It helps us help you.

SKIN CONCERN OVER SKIN TYPE: YOUR ROADMAP TO BRIGHT, CLEAR SKIN

Skin is dynamic, changing with the seasons, stress, hormones and the simple passage of time.

Throughout this chapter, I've challenged a skincare belief that has long been held sacred – that your skin type is the most important factor in selecting skincare. The reality, as we've seen, is far more nuanced and rigidly sticking to a skin-type-based approach to skincare won't always serve you well.

Instead, addressing your skin concerns directly allows you to understand and adapt to your skin's needs in real time. This approach is inherently flexible, responsive and powerful. It allows your skincare routine to evolve gracefully with you, through every stage of life. Understanding your skin through its concerns empowers you, liberating you from marketing-driven 'categories' and myths that keep you stuck.

As we turn to the next chapters, you'll learn exactly how to build your concern-focused skincare routine. We'll explore the standout ingredients that deliver real, tangible improvements and how to thoughtfully combine them in a supportive routine that respects your skin's innate sensitivity.

Armed with this deeper understanding, you're now ready to take control. It's time to move beyond traditional labels and embrace a smarter, more personalized path to great skincare.

4

Getting Back to Basics

SKINCARE OVERWHELM

I took to YouTube in 2015 almost entirely because of one specific problem. I was seeing droves of (mostly) women in my clinic who had what I called 'London Skin'.

The symptoms were striking: an irritable, bumpy, breakout-prone complexion concealed beneath a thick layer of longwear make-up. The more they did to their skin, the more it misbehaved. It wasn't uncommon for someone to arrive at my consulting rooms with a suitcase filled with products, clearly having spent a heap of cash, utterly lost as to why their skin was so unhappy.

This coincided with the rise of a new generation of direct-to-consumer skincare brands that built viral followings by democratizing access to active ingredients, bringing what had previously been the preserve of the dermatologist's or aesthetician's office to a mass audience at a fraction of the price.

The problem was that many of these high-strength, single-use actives were launched with minimal guidance, assuming a level of scientific literacy that most consumers – and, crucially, creators – simply didn't have. There was no expert at the wheel when it came to diagnosis or routine-building. Instead, well-meaning amateurs shared their skincare routines from the comfort of their living rooms. This wasn't intentional; no one could have predicted the influence or reach of the early YouTubers. Yet they went on to shape the behaviour of a generation of beauty-loving men and women. A relentless conveyor belt of newness turned the everyday beauty routine into a status symbol, as the pendulum swung away from function and into the realm of cult.

Many of the patients I was seeing were in thrall to the trend for elaborate 10-step Korean skincare routines that were being shared by their favourite influencers. Oil-based double cleansing (a two-step cleansing routine using an oil to dissolve sunscreen and make-up followed by a water-based cleanser to get all the oil off) was a constant in these rituals, as were exfoliating toners and cocktailing actives.

It was a formative time for me; I honed my craft in removing complexity from skincare routines for my patients. Recognizing that this was a bigger problem, I started to share my clinic protocols with my audience online. Ultimately, they became the basis for Dr Sam's Skincare and it's that very underpinning philosophy I want to share with you here.

THE COMPLEXITY TRAP

What happens when your skin barrier isn't facing a one-off assault, but rather a daily siege?

In Chapter 3, we saw how a single harsh product or environmental challenge can breach your skin's barrier walls, causing the acute inflammation we call irritant dermatitis. This is where a chronic damage pattern develops. When you subject your skin barrier to constant, low-level attacks (morning acid toner and vitamin C, evening retinol, then weekend exfoliant), each individual assault might seem manageable. But faced with a relentless onslaught, the walls need to be constantly repaired and never fully regain their strength. Your skin's repair crew, the dutiful keratinocytes, become exhausted. They're so busy patching up the damage of the day that they can't reinforce for tomorrow's challenges.

What starts as trying to 'optimize' your routine becomes a cycle where you keep adding in more actives when your skin needs a break.

THE COST OF OVERTREATMENT

Despite your skin's inherent brilliance, it does need daily maintenance to preserve the strength and function of its walls and ensure the health of the local residents. That's where your skincare routine comes in. Like a trusted construction crew, the best team shows up consistently, uses reliable materials and makes measured, thoughtful repairs. Now, picture a crew run by an erratic foreman – he switches from limestone on Monday, to sandstone on Tuesday, then to steel by Wednesday. Each material might be excellent in isolation, but together? They create an inconsistent patchwork, strong in some spots, weak in others. Over time, the city walls suffer.

If you've ever subscribed to a beauty box, that's exactly what happens. When we constantly change up our skincare products, piling on a random selection of newness – serums, essences, toners – without a clear purpose, it can easily overwhelm the skin, eroding its integrity and disrupting the delicate balance of its microbiome. It exposes skin to an ever-changing barrage of new preservatives, varying pH and actives.

A healthy microbiome is like a diverse, multicultural neighbourhood.

A healthy microbiome is like a diverse, multicultural neighbourhood – different species of bacteria working together, each filling important roles. Product switching reduces this diversity – a vibrant community becomes a bland row of identical chain stores.

As a consequence, the reliable interaction between our microbiome and the immune system is disrupted, interrupting a vital educational channel where our friendly residents send chemical messages that help reassure the immune system that all is well. Your immune system becomes confused, more reactive and more likely to sound false alarms when faced with perfectly innocent ingredients. This is why product switching often leads to increased sensitivity and breakouts, rather than the glowing skin you were promised on social media.

Each sensitivity reaction creates more inflammation, which further compromises your barrier, which makes you more sensitive to the next product... It's a vicious cycle that many people find themselves trapped in, wondering why their skin has become so tricky, when they're trying so hard to take care of it.

YOUR SKIN IS CRYING OUT FOR SIMPLICITY

I have lost count of the number of times I've been hailed as a miracle worker – and it's all because of my red pen. Every new patient I see completes a form detailing their history and, crucially, what they're currently using on their skin. These lists often require supplementary pages to accommodate the full list of potions in rotation. I learned to spot patterns based on their choice of products ('ah, you must follow xxx'). This information was extremely helpful, as I then knew what philosophy I might have to challenge.

Invariably, at least 90 per cent of it had to go. I'd choose the appropriate actives based on their skin concern and then suggest a simple support system to work alongside them. If they had sensitive skin, I'd often suggest a gap between starting the support products and then subsequently adding in the actives, so that we knew what was doing what. It wasn't uncommon to get an email at about two weeks in, saying their skin had done a complete U-turn. How was this possible? There was no medicine involved! Such is the power of simplification and a ruthless edit. After all, the first tenet of being a doctor is 'do no harm'.

The truth is that your skin is crying out for consistency because that's how it's designed to function. Like any complex system, it craves homeostasis, performing best when it can establish routines, build on stable foundations, helping maintain equilibrium.

The irony is almost comical – in our quest to optimize our skin, we've become the architects of the very problems we're trying to solve. The solution isn't more products, stronger actives, or more frequent treatments. It's stepping back, letting your skin's physiology get back into balance, and then working with it, rather than against it.

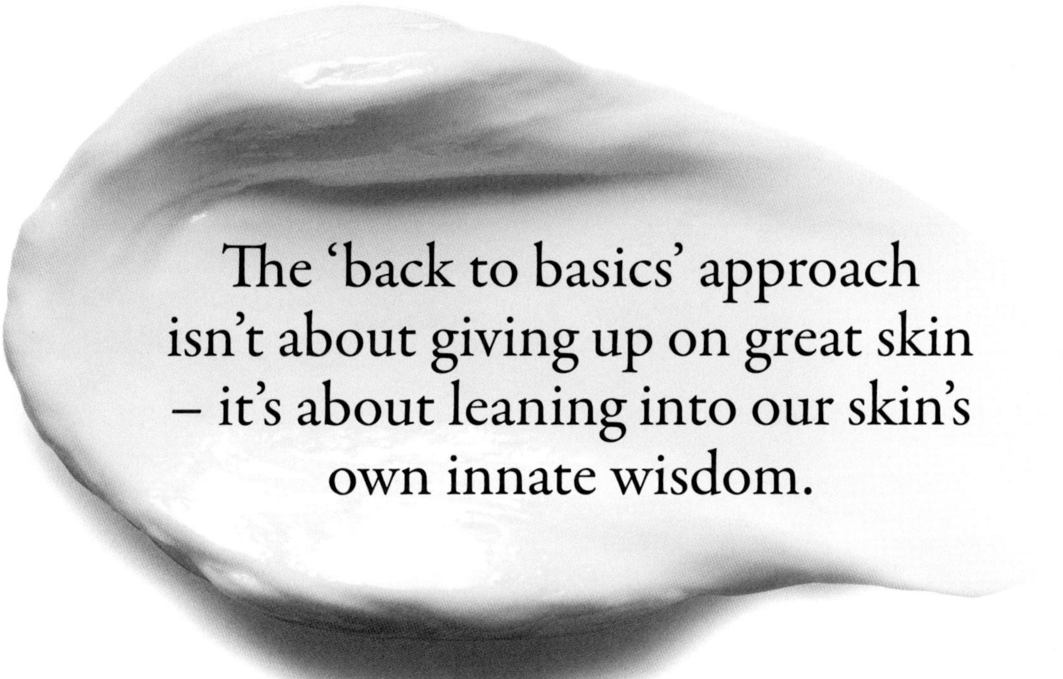

BUILDING YOUR SKINCARE FOUNDATIONS: THE FOUR PILLAR FRAMEWORK

Making friends with your skin barrier is the crux of a basic skincare routine.

We dare not introduce actives until we have made friends with our skin barrier. If you try to transform skin overnight with a retinoid when you haven't done barrier maintenance, the walls will come crumbling down.

So, let me introduce you to the framework that will change everything: **The Four Pillars**. This is a strategic approach that ensures that every product in your routine has a clear purpose and works in harmony with the others. It's the basis of every clinic protocol I've ever built for my patients.

THE FOUR PILLARS

1	**Cleanse** (see opposite)
2	**Activate** (see page 81)
3	**Hydrate** (see page 81)
4	**Protect** (see page 83)

1 CLEANSE

Cleansing is the first pillar of any good skincare routine. However, it comes with a built-in tension. The goal is simple: remove the things you *don't* want on your skin (oil, make-up, pollution, sunscreen) without stripping away the elements that keep it healthy, hydrated and resilient. Remember that even something as innocent as splashing your face with tap water erodes your skin barrier, taking just a little of the mortar out from between the bricks.

We must also be mindful of our skin's acid mantle (see page 27). This natural defence film deters troublesome microbes from moving in by ensuring friendly ones stay put. Aggressive cleansing is the single most common cause of acid mantle disruption, leading to dryness, irritation and intolerant skin.

Every cleanser ultimately works in the same way: they use surfactants **(1)**. These are molecules with split personalities – an oil-loving side and a water-loving side. The oily bit grabs onto the grime/make-up **(2, 3)** and the water-soluble bit allows water to wash it away **(4)**. The challenge is that surfactants can't tell the difference between what needs to be removed and what doesn't. That's why cleansing in the most minimal fashion wins every time.

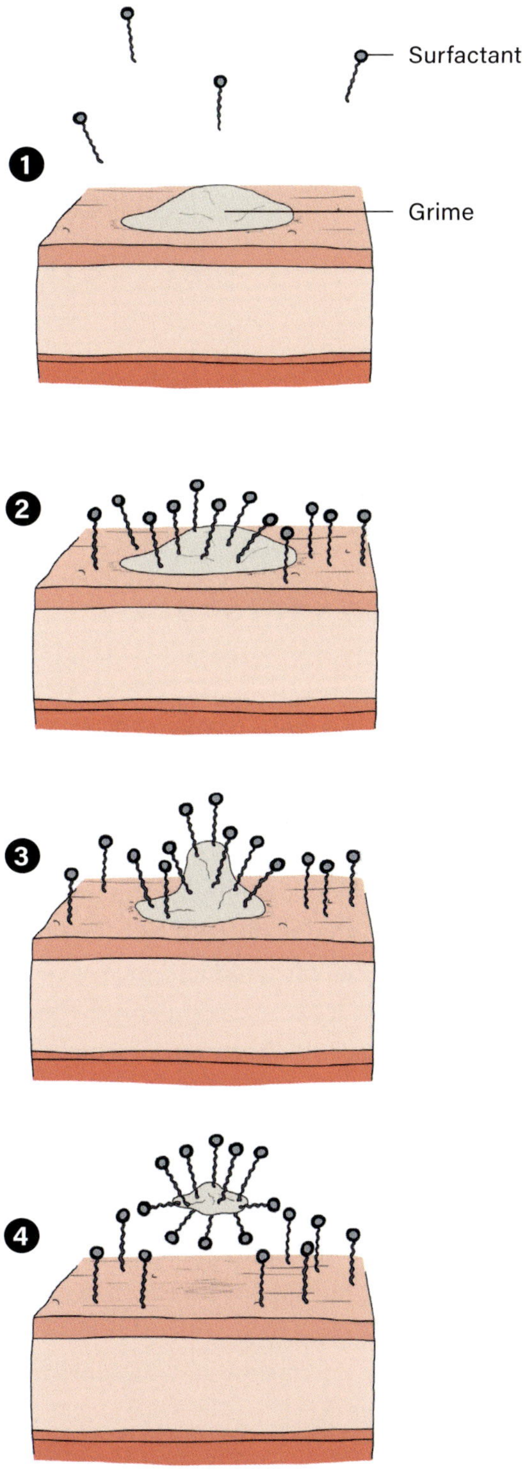

HOW CLEANSER WORKS

Take the fewest actions necessary to clean the skin.

TO FOAM OR NOT TO FOAM

I took a stance early in my career that has continued to cause provocation to this day: to ditch foaming cleansers altogether from my practice.

The poster child for foaming surfactants is Sodium Lauryl Sulphate (or SLS). SLS is found in many personal care products, such as cleansers and shampoos. It became popular as far back as the 1930s because it was cheap to formulate with and consumers associated the rich, satisfying foam (which removed oil enthusiastically) with efficacy and cleanliness. That squeaky-clean feeling provided immediate sensory reward. Alas, the squeak is a red flag. SLS can damage the skin barrier by pulling out too much of the lipid mortar. At the same time, it's hard to rinse away, disrupting the acid mantle and microbiome. Hello, sensitive skin!

The good news is that not all surfactants foam. While SLS lathers because of chemical charges that render it anionic (negatively charged), we can instead choose gentle, non-charged surfactants that are innately kinder to your skin barrier. Their target market is those with sensitive skin, but I find that once you educate people on the idea that a cleanser doesn't need to foam to clean, they actually suit almost everyone.

Next comes the question of whether or not our cleanser needs assistance to be effective. Let me come back to the idea of doing no harm – we want to take the fewest actions necessary to clean the skin. My policy is to use nothing rougher than fingertips to aid the cleansing process. Anything beyond this adds an abrasive element, so I discourage the use of flannels, cloths and cleansing devices. This is especially true for those with a sensitive skin issue, such as rosacea.

AVOID ACTIVES IN YOUR CLEANSER

I do not recommend the use of actives *in* your cleanser. There are two reasons:

Firstly, they increase its irritation factor and invariably end up in the delicate eye area, which dries the thin, delicate skin unnecessarily. Exfoliating acids do not belong in the eye area.

Secondly, there's no way of controlling how much of the active you might be receiving. Given how little time a cleanser spends on your skin, invariably most of it is going to wind up going down the plughole.

It is better to skip actives in your cleanser altogether and administer them in the form of a leave-on product, which you can dose and distribute accurately.

DOES IT MATTER WHERE YOU CLEANSE?

The temperature of the water you use to cleanse matters, but the location of the cleanse does not. I have always cleansed in the shower in the morning – it makes it easy to rinse your skin thoroughly. I simply ensure I cleanse after I've used haircare products (to ensure all residue from the hairline is removed) and I adjust the water so it's tepid. Hot water strips out more mortar than tepid water, depleting your skin barrier, so we want to avoid that.

MORNING CLEANSE: YAY OR NAY?

For the vast majority of people, a morning cleanse is advised to remove oil and dead skin cells. As 65 per cent of us have combination skin, that means there's oil in our T-zone that needs to be removed every morning. Sebum blocks penetration of many skincare products, so it's helpful to remove it from both a functional point of view as well as for simple aesthetics.

The exception is those with dry skin. In the absence of visible oil on the skin's surface, splashing skin with water in the morning might well be all you need. A cleanse in the evening is always recommended to remove pollution (which drives pigmentation), dead skin cells and whatever products have been on your skin during the day.

NOTES FROM THE CLINIC

Before Dr Sam's was born, I recommended non-foaming gel cleansers from French pharmacy brands to my patients, but when they were repeatedly discontinued or reformulated, I took matters into my own hands and created Flawless Cleanser. Many years later, the formula remains unchanged. It does exactly what a cleanser is supposed to do – no more, no less – and it's suitable for almost everyone, whatever their skin concern.

AVOID DOUBLE CLEANSING

I do not recommend double cleansing. I believe that a single cleanse, correctly performed with the right type of cleanser should suffice. If you're wearing the kind of make-up on your skin where this feels like a necessity (such as longwear, 18-hour or similar), my advice is to adjust this practice rather than double cleanse.

Often, the reason for wearing longwear make-up is because of the security it offers, which is understandable in the face of punishing, unpredictable breakouts, for example. Blemishes and pigmentation hidden beneath are reliably concealed. However, the paradox is that many of these formulas are occlusive to pores, perpetuating the problem. Meanwhile, elaborate cleansing can aggravate the skin barrier and actually worsen breakouts.

Working backwards from the issue, if we correct these problems with actives (the root-cause approach), over time we reduce the need for longwear coverage. This then allows for less complicated cleansing, which allows for a stronger barrier and more space for powerful actives . . . and so a virtuous cycle is set up that leads towards increasingly bright, clear skin. That is what I want for you. Then, make-up becomes an optional tool of enhancement, rather than a necessary cloak to hide behind. It's much more fun. It's also half the cost.

2 ACTIVATE

If the word 'active' is new to you, here's what it means: an ingredient that delivers a specific biological effect inside your cells. Not on the surface. *Inside.* That's why they have the power to transform.

Using active ingredients is where things get very exciting! BUT it deserves a chapter of its own. So, I'm going to keep you on the edge of your seat until the next chapter (see pages 89–119). It's *that* important.

3 HYDRATE

If cleansing is removing grime and graffiti from your city's walls, hydration (moisturizing) is repairing the mortar between the bricks. This allows the skin to remain a largely impenetrable barrier, so unwanted things don't get in. It also helps your skin hold on to just the right amount of water, so it doesn't all escape into the atmosphere. This keeps skin flexible yet resilient, but also ensures organized exfoliation of the wall's bricks, allowing them to completely renew every 28 days.

Moisturizers work through three main types of ingredients: occlusives, humectants and emollients. Each plays a different role in helping the skin stay supple and comfortable.

OCCLUSIVES: LOCKING WATER IN

Occlusives form a physical seal on the surface of the skin and prevent evaporation of water, just like clingfilm does for your dinner in the refrigerator. This function is particularly helpful for dry or compromised skin that loses water quickly, especially in challenging cold or dry climates. They work best when applied to damp skin. Commonly used occlusives include shea butter, silicones such as dimethicone, and mineral oil.

HUMECTANTS: DRAWING WATER IN

These are ingredients such as glycerin, hyaluronic acid and urea, which act like water magnets. They attract water from one of two directions into the stratum corneum, either from the environment on the outside or from the deeper layers of the skin on the inside. Think of them as sponges that soak up and hold on to moisture where it's needed. This helps to increase water content in the upper layers of the skin, making it look plump, feel soft and move flexibly.

There is a catch. Water will always try to move from an area of high concentration to one of low concentration by osmosis, so if the air is dry and cold, moisture will move from the deeper layers of the skin (where water is more plentiful) to the surface of the skin and then evaporate into the air, leaving it parched. This is not what we want. However, there is a work-around – and it's why humectants are almost always formulated with occlusives. This combination allows water to be drawn into the stratum corneum, keeping it supple, and then trapped there safely by the occlusive. This isn't an issue if the atmosphere is warm and humid – think holiday in Hawaii – as moisture will flow in the opposite direction, from the air into the outer layer of the skin, keeping it juicy.

EMOLLIENTS: FILLING THE GAPS

These make our skin softer, by smoothing the surface. They fill in the gaps between skin cells – the mortar in our wall – using lipids. Some of them are also occlusives, reducing the escape of water through the skin barrier. Silicones are both emollients and occlusives whereas isopropyl palmitate is an emollient only.

In an ideal world, proper hydration will utilize all three types of ingredients to rebuild the skin's barrier, reduce water loss, and help the skin feel smooth and function optimally. Just like cleansing, this is a critical component of daily maintenance. It's essential we've got this right before we even think about our next step.

4 PROTECT

I've already put my stake in the ground on the subject of wearing sunscreen daily (see page 20). But how do we choose the right one? There are four key pieces of information on a sunscreen bottle to consider when making your choice.

1 SPF

This is the Sun Protection Factor and it's a measure of the duration of defence it provides against burning UVB rays. You can think of it as a multiplier of time. If your skin typically burns after 10 minutes of being exposed to the sun, then SPF30 theoretically protects you for 10 minutes × 30, i.e. 300 minutes (5 hours).

That sounds quite a lot, right? But in practice, no sunscreen reliably stays on the skin perfectly intact for that long. Many become less effective over time, because UV rays cause the filters to break down and sweat and friction from clothing or towel use means coverage becomes patchy. For these reasons, reapplication every two hours when in direct sunlight is recommended.

More usefully in practice, the SPF gives us information on the level of protection against UVB rays (its filtration power).

See the diagram below. That 1 per cent difference between SPF30 and SPF50 might not seem like much. But SPF30 lets through 50% more UV radiation than SPF50. Over a lifetime that difference stacks up.

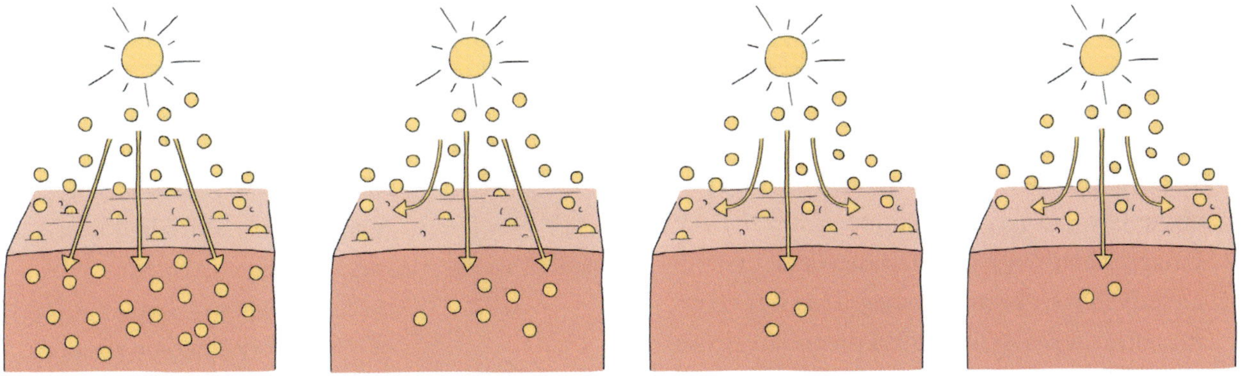

SPF0
0% UVB rays blocked

SPF15
93% UVB rays blocked

SPF30
97% UVB rays blocked

SPF50
98% UVB rays blocked

2 UVA PROTECTION

UVA doesn't cause burning, but it's the driving force behind premature ageing and pigmentation, and contributes to skin cancer, so it's just as important to protect the skin from it. The first thing to look for on the label is the term 'broad spectrum'. That tells us it blocks both UVA and UVB rays. How much UVA protection is present is demonstrated in a number of ways, depending on where in the world your sunscreen was formulated.

- **EU and UK:** UVA in a circle symbol means that the sunscreen offers *at least* one-third of the level of UVA protection as that of UVB protection. So an SPF30 has at least a UVA protection factor of 10. This is considered the most reliable and consistent system in use.

- **Asia:** UVA protection is denoted by the PA rating (Protection Grade of UVA) and graded + to ++++. This is based on a lab protocol called the Persistent Pigment Darkening (PPD) test, which measures how long UVA exposure takes to trigger tanning in skin with and without the sunscreen (I talked about UVA triggering an immediate tan back in Chapter 2 through UVA oxidation of melanin already in your keratinocytes). That is used to measure the *strength* of UVA protection in an SPF. The PPD test result is then translated into a PA+ rating. In essence, the more +, the stronger the UVA rating.

- **US:** The UVA labelling system is limited to stating that a sunscreen is broad spectrum – that's it. That means it blocks UVA up to what's known as the critical wavelength (370nm). The issue with this is that it doesn't tell us how strongly it does this, just how broadly. It also doesn't tell us about how it protects against the longer wavelengths of UVA beyond 370nm, which are especially important in those with darker skin tones and melasma. This means there is much greater variability in the level of UVA protection offered, so it's harder to gauge their effectiveness. This is probably a consequence of the very limited number of UVA sunscreen filters the FDA have approved for use in the US.

3 WATER RESISTANCE

If claimed, the label should state: water-resistant to 40 or 80 minutes. This means the sunscreen maintains its stated SPF for that duration while swimming or sweating, but not indefinitely.

4 APPLICATION AND REAPPLICATION GUIDANCE

A responsible SPF label should include guidance on how to use the sunscreen to achieve the level of protection stated on the pack (see page 130).

MINERAL VS CHEMICAL

A sunscreen filter is the ingredient that blocks UV rays. The chemical structure of a sunscreen filter determines what bit of the UV spectrum it will absorb – some like UVA and some like UVB. The best sunscreens combine several filters to give full, balanced protection.

Chemical sunscreens use filters such as octinoxate or oxybenzone, which absorb UV rays and convert them into harmless energy, preventing DNA damage in your skin. They are brilliant for everyday use due to their cosmetic elegance and exceptional long-wave UVA1 cover (for example, Tinosorb and Mexoryl). They can be formulated into a lightweight shield that layers well and won't leave a visible cast.

Mineral (or physical) sunscreens rely on ingredients such as zinc oxide and titanium dioxide, which sit on the surface of the skin to reflect and scatter UV light, while also absorbing part of it. Again, they're working to neutralize the sun's rays before they can land on your skin and do harm. If your skin is sensitive, redness-prone, or affected by rosacea or eczema, a mineral formula will work well. They're also ideal after treatments such as lasers or micro-needling, when your skin barrier needs extra protection, and they tend not to sting the eyes.

UV ISN'T THE WHOLE STORY

Visible light also has a role to play in how our skin ages. These longer wavelengths are lower in energy but much greater in number than UV rays. Blue light is a particular consideration when tackling pigmentation (see Chapter 2, page 30), especially in darker skin tones. It also plays a role in generating ROS (see page 40) and driving premature ageing. Using a sunscreen containing iron oxides to block visible light is thus helpful, especially given that it offers useful cosmetic benefits at the same time – it's the pigment found in foundations and concealers. A good colour match to skin tone is key.

HOW DO YOU CHOOSE?

This can all sound a little overwhelming, so here's what I tell my patients: use broad-spectrum SPF50 for daily use and choose one that's labelled PA++++ or has the symbol UVA in a circle.

We want the maximum UVA protection for everyday use because UVA rays are the sneaky ones present all year round that age us. We know we're unlikely to burn from UVB exposure in January in the UK, so the SPF bit is redundant then. But we *are* susceptible to aging every day of the year, thanks to UVA. The way to get high UVA protection is through using broad-spectrum, high-factor sunscreen that's quantified on the pack.

Beyond that, I recommend those with darker skin tones use a sunscreen with a tint for the additional blue light protection. Choose one with a texture you love, so that it's a pleasure to be used daily and layers well with the rest of your morning routine. That makes it a keeper.

You may even want to have a couple of different sunscreens for different uses. A great sunscreen is a bit like a perfect pair of jeans – there's one for every occasion and the right fit can change everything.

IDEAL SUNSCREENS FOR YOUR SKIN CONCERN

- **Acne-prone:** Won't clog pores (labelled non-comedogenic).
- **Melasma:** Long-wave UVA protection, tinted, water-resistant in summer.
- **Eczema:** Mineral-based.
- **Rosacea-prone:** Mineral-based (especially if you have ocular rosacea), tinted.

KEY FEATURES OF A SUN HAT

- A 7-cm (2¾-inch) brim.
- A UPF* of 50.
- Made of a tightly woven, coloured fabric.
- Collapsible, so it can be easily tossed in your bag (having it to hand is key).

** UPF (Ultraviolet Protection Factor) is equivalent to SPF, but for clothing.*

MY PERSONAL ROUTINE

As someone firmly on the rosacea spectrum, I wear a tinted mineral SPF50 sunscreen on WFH days. It allows me to top up easily through the day, makes me look pulled together without the need to wear make-up and doesn't sting my eyes if I work out. On my more polished days, I wear an untinted SPF50 sunscreen that primes nicely under make-up. I avoid UV exposure later on in the day, as I won't reapply.

The Four Pillar structure has served my patients and me well over the last two decades. Simplification doesn't just help your skin; it also reduces the cognitive load and decision fatigue around your skincare choices. Too many products, leading to skin barrier breakdown and microbiome malaise, are so often the hidden culprits behind sensitive skin. The solution is doing less, but better. Master these steps and you'll create the foundations of a strong, impactful routine. This sets the scene for the magic of actives, allowing you to unlock true transformation without sacrificing your skin's integrity.

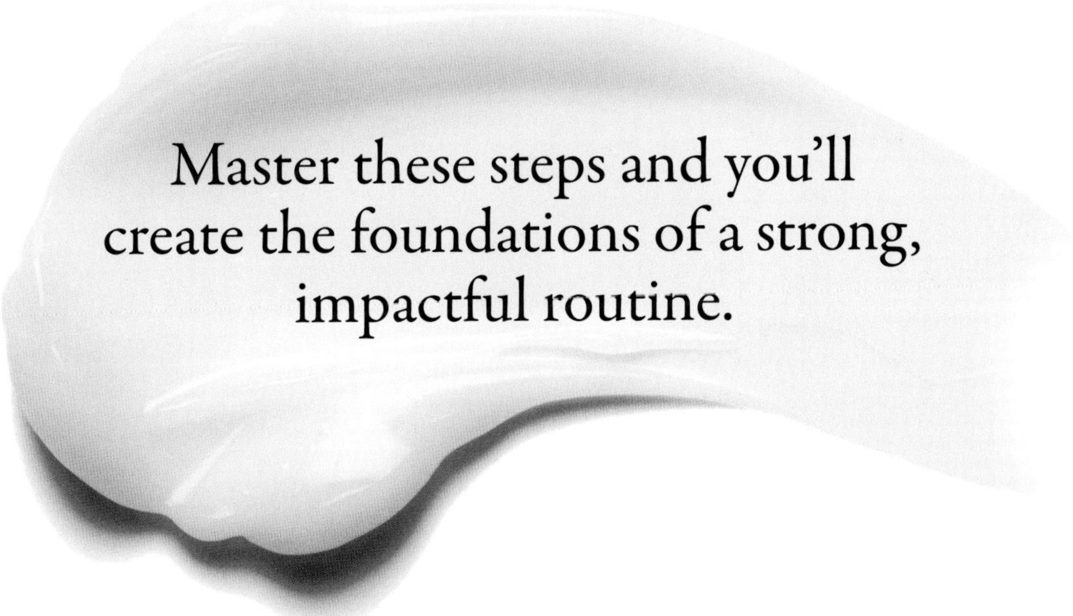

Master these steps and you'll create the foundations of a strong, impactful routine.

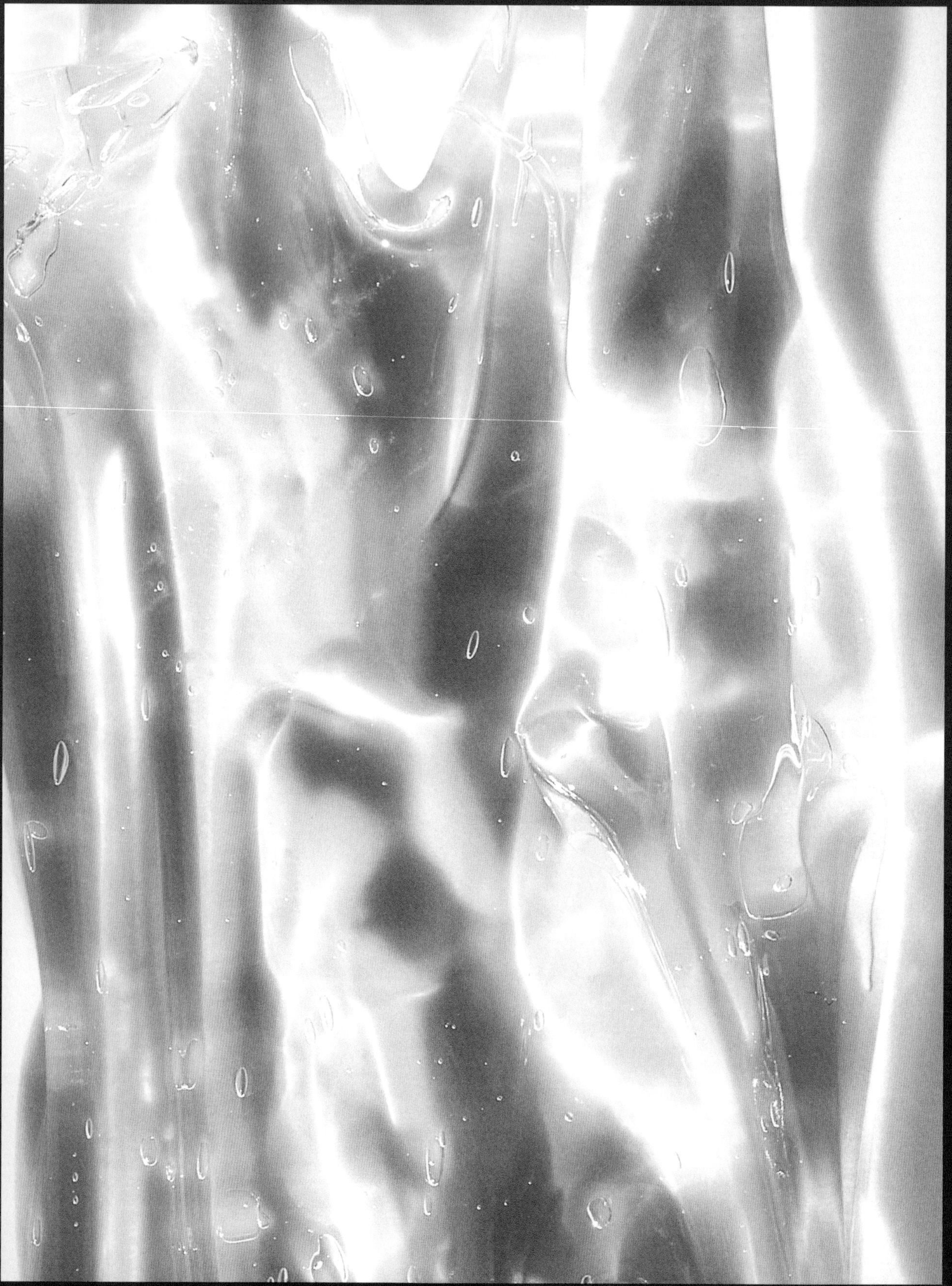

5

Demystifying Active Ingredients

INTRODUCING ACTIVES

You've built your foundations, now you're ready to enter the realm of transformation. This is where active ingredients are waiting to work their magic.

Admittedly the world of actives can seem incredibly intimidating. Ampoules! Essences! Boosters! The names alone are enough to make you roll your eyes and tune out. So let me make one thing clear: it's not about the name on the front of the bottle; it's about what's inside it. What truly matters is this: a formula with the *right ingredients*, in the *right combination*, at the *right concentration* matched to *your* specific skin goals.

Using actives well is a skill I've mastered over the years, blending that geeky early interest in pharmacology with hands-on clinical experience. I've seen what works and what doesn't. Once you know what to look for, the noise falls away and you'll only ever buy what your skin actually needs.

WHAT IS AN ACTIVE INGREDIENT?

If you're new to skincare, an active ingredient might be an alien concept to you. What I mean by the term 'active' is an ingredient that goes beyond simply supporting your skin. Instead, it delivers a specific biological effect, for example stimulating collagen production.

Most actives work through actions *inside* the cell, as opposed to working externally. This is fundamental to why they're so effective – they are changing how your cells behave. You'll learn how the most useful actives tend to be multitaskers, with several targets within the cell, hence their versatility in helping solve different concerns.

The active skincare space has become rather muddled, because you can now find actives in everything, even cleansers and sunscreens. But I am a reductionist. I believe we get the best results when we create a dedicated slot in our routine for these actives. We can then treat them scientifically, dosing them accurately and distributing them precisely. Then we measure and track the results. These are the hallmarks of actives well used.

This approach allows you to see the fruits of your labour, so it becomes clear when you need to alter the strategy to move closer to your desired goal.

GOAL SETTING

Before you set off on your actives voyage, you need to make a plan. What are your goals and what is the starting point? We need some structure, otherwise it's exceedingly easy to be lured off course.

- One of the best methods for this is to take some barefaced selfies to document your starting point. Always take your selfies in the same location at the same time of day, so that the lighting is as consistent as possible.
- Review your progress at sensible intervals – every 6 weeks is a good idea initially, as this is about one skin cycle (the time it takes for your epidermis to renew).
- Finally, put your plan into writing. The bathroom mirror is a good place to pin it.

All of these actions make it easy to remember your intentions from the outset.

So how do you know what active or actives you need? And at what strength? In this chapter I will share with you the actives I use on a daily basis, focusing on the top six – the ride-or-die ones, without which I couldn't practise. This narrow lens forces real consideration of how they act and indeed interact with each other. I'll then share with you my honourable mentions – some might be newer to my toolkit, others simply get used less frequently. You'll see how it all comes together.

NOTES FROM THE CLINIC

I had one patient who took the planning part of the process so seriously, she created an Excel spreadsheet of her skincare plan after our first meeting. Needless to say, she was able to follow the plan to the letter and her new skincare habits quickly became programmed into her subconscious without effort. Of course, this is not for everyone. Build your habit in a way that sets you up to win. It's said that we need around two months for a daily habit to become automatic. Make it easy by doing your skincare routine after brushing your teeth morning and night.

MY TOP SIX ACTIVES

1	**Retinoids** (see opposite)
2	**Azelaic acid** (see page 99)
3	**Niacinamide** (see page 103)
4	**Salicylic acid** (see page 106)
5	**Benzoyl peroxide** (see page 109)
6	**Vitamin C** (see page 112)

ALSO FEATURED **(SEE PAGE 118)**

- Bakuchiol
- Lactic acid
- Hydroquinone

1 RETINOIDS

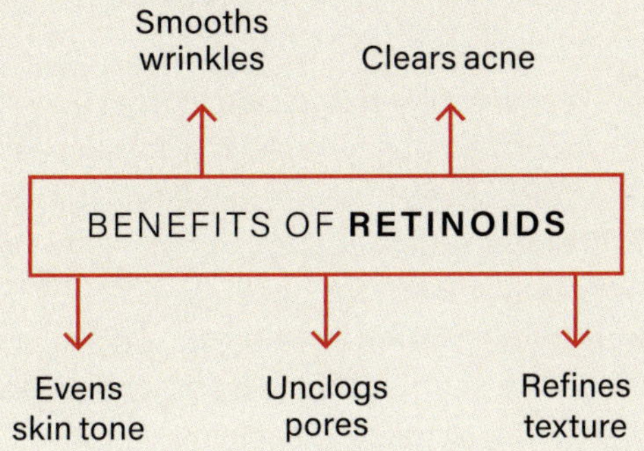

I'm commencing the discussion of actives with the most important category of all: retinoids. They are considered the gold standard of all the actives when it comes to tackling the signs of ageing.

Any conversation about actives has to start here. I can tell if someone is using a retinoid from across the room: that's how impactful they are. But they are also the active that can trigger a tremendous amount of fear. I'm here to show you the upside of using one and help dispel that fear. I believe that almost everyone **can** and **should** use a retinoid.

The principles of how we start using a retinoid can be applied to almost all actives.

WHAT ARE THEY?

A retinoid is the name for the group of ingredients derived from vitamin A. Retinoids are brilliant for preserving youthful skin, managing breakouts, unclogging pores and fading pigmentation.

The list includes, but is not limited to:

Non-prescription (meaning they are classed as a cosmetic): retinol, retinaldehyde, retinyl palmitate/propionate, retinyl retinoate, hydroxypinacolone retinoate (HPR)

Prescription (meaning they are classed as a drug because they are significantly more potent and a doctor needs to prescribe them): adapalene, tretinoin, tazarotene, trifarotene

RETINOID	POTENCY
Tazarotene	High
All-trans retinoic acid (tretinoin)	
Trifarotene	
Adapalene	Medium
Hydroxypinacolone retinoate	
Retinaldehyde (retinal)	
Retinol	Low
Retinyl palmitate	Very Low

HOW THEY WORK

It is hard to grasp that just one ingredient can do all of the following: increase collagen production, reduce collagen breakdown, drive faster cell turnover in the epidermis and more even melanin distribution, stimulate new blood vessels in the dermis, prevent clumping of keratinocytes in the hair follicles . . . There is little that isn't influenced by a retinoid when it comes to skin health.

Our skin is full of receptors for retinoids. A receptor is basically a lock and, in this instance, the retinoid is the key. When the retinoid unlocks its dedicated receptor, it switches on the expression of genes. When I tell you that retinoids influence over 3000 genes in your skin, does that not blow your mind? For context, we have about 20,000 genes in total, in every single cell in our body. Of these, 15,000 of them are active in your skin. So we are influencing 20 per cent of your skin's active genetic material *with a product you apply to your skin.* I get a bit misty-eyed when I think about the ways a retinoid affects your skin. That's because their actions so profoundly change our skin for the better. When we use a retinoid, we are tapping into a built-in blueprint for healthy and beautiful skin, even when we're trying to correct a disease process like acne. Such is their power.

WHAT THEY TREAT

Retinoids were first harnessed to treat acne, because of their ability to stop sticky skin cells gluing themselves together in the hair follicles, thus preventing comedone formation, the root cause of why blemishes occur (see page 48). They were also found to help get rid of existing comedones, soothe inflammation and speed up cell turnover, tackling acne in several additional checkpoints in its evolution.

Retinoids dramatically improved the outcome for acne sufferers who then remained on treatment long term for preventative reasons. Clinicians at follow-up noted that their patients were ageing rather beautifully. Upon further exploration, individuals had fewer lines, less pigmentation and smoother skin texture – a 'rosy glow' to the complexion was noted.

Retinoids have been studied more than any other skincare ingredient and are considered the gold standard for treating photo-ageing. They've been found to be helpful in the treatment of everything from melasma to rosacea, and even acne scarring.

HOW TO CHOOSE

A common challenge is knowing which one to go for and at what strength. Many retinoids are marketed at a vast number of different strengths.

Not all retinoids arrive ready to work; some need to undergo a conversion process that relies on enzymes in your skin cells, and the process is inefficient – only a fraction of what you apply ever reaches the active form retinoic acid; and what's produced tends to arrive in bursts rather than steadily, which drives irritation.

Retinol, the form found in most over-the-counter products, requires two conversion steps before it can bind to retinoid receptors and take effect. Retinaldehyde requires just one, making it more efficient, though it can still cause irritation in its own right.

Tretinoin is retinoic acid: it binds directly, no conversion needed, which is why tretinoin at 0.1% is twenty times stronger than retinol at the same concentration. Hydroxypinacolone retinoate (HPR) is different again. It also binds directly to retinoid receptors without need for conversion (albeit at lower potency than tretinoin), making it efficient, with excellent tolerability.

I mostly use prescription tretinoin in my clinic and three strengths of this have sufficed over two decades of clinical practice. In the non-prescription space, I like HPR. I recommend 2% HPR to start with and 5% when you're tolerant to 2%. If that gets you to your goals, super. Stop there. If not, go to see a dermatologist and get prescription tretinoin and work up the strengths until you reach your threshold for tolerance or you reach your goal.

HOW FAST YOU'LL SEE RESULTS

Results start as early as 4–6 weeks into use, as the quality of the epidermis improves under their influence. More meaningful changes to the dermis require the building of proteins, so will take longer. You can expect to see fine lines and wrinkles improve over 3–6 months. When I tell you that these improvements will continue beyond 12 months and longer, it's no exaggeration.

WORD OF WARNING

Retinoids are not for everyone – avoid them during pregnancy (see page 141), or if you have active eczema or rosacea.

COMMON RETINOID MYTHS

Retinoids are the source of more myths than any other active skincare ingredient. So pernicious are these myths that they've even discouraged some of the most experienced beauty editors. I have sympathy for anyone with this job, as it requires them to change their skincare on an almost daily basis to test out the ever-increasing deluge of new skincare products. It's unsurprising I see so many of them with skin issues – it's high-risk work.

1 Retinoids thin the skin

This might be *the* top retinoid myth. The reality is that retinoids make your dermis thicker, which is exactly what we want. Retinoids stimulate more collagen production, which means a more wrinkle-resistant complexion. This is a very good thing. They do make the stratum corneum of the epidermis temporarily thinner and more compactly packed, but again this is actually beneficial, not damaging. It improves texture and glow. So, we can firmly put this myth to bed.

2 You can't use retinoids if you have sensitive skin

Sensitive skin can certainly benefit from retinoids, providing introduction is slow and the correct level of potency is chosen. I'm a huge fan of HPR in this instance. It delivers excellent efficacy with relatively little irritation. Barrier support from the rest of your routine is, naturally, key. This myth has deterred many who would benefit (for example, those with rosacea-prone skin), who often do very well with a low-dose retinoid once their skin is under control.

3 You shouldn't use retinoids in summer

It's absolutely fine to continue using your retinoid through summer. They do not render skin more sun-sensitive (quite the opposite, in fact). Of course, it's sensible to observe the rules of sun safety alongside your retinoid, as we are striving to prevent the consequences of UV exposure.

Make sure you have a high-factor, broad-spectrum SPF and apply it in the correct quantity. Wear a proper hat (see box, page 86), avoid the strong hours of the sun between 11am and 3pm, and reapply SPF every two hours. If you're doing all this consistently, continuing with your retinoid is fine. Plenty of people living in hot countries all year round manage this perfectly well. Skipping your retinoid all summer will set your progress back substantially, especially if you're using it for acne management.

4 Retinoids exfoliate the skin

Retinoids improve skin texture, but by a different mechanism to classic exfoliation. Physical scrubs and chemical exfoliants, such as alpha hydroxy acids, work by disrupting the bonds between skin cells *on the outside*. This removes the top layer of our skin to reveal smoother, brighter cells underneath. Retinoids work *on the inside* at a deeper, regenerative level by switching on genes that speed up cell turnover and by changing the way our skin cells differentiate. They improve the blueprint for building a strong, organized wall, rather than simply knocking some worn-out bricks off the top.

5 You have to purge before seeing results

The idea of purging, with more breakouts in the early stages of treatment, puts a lot of acne sufferers off starting a retinoid when they would undoubtedly benefit. This happens because the retinoid encourages all existing clogged pores to push through in a synchronized manner, so it can make the skin get temporarily worse, as it brings things to the surface.

In reality, it doesn't always happen. Using an anti-inflammatory will help make it more bearable (see salicylic acid, pages 106–8, and benzoyl peroxide, pages 109–11). But if it does, I ask patients to look at it like this: instead of getting your allotted number of blemishes over the next 6 months, you'll get them over the next 2–6 weeks, but then the retinoid's continued influence will prevent the pores from clogging up again. On the other side of the purging, lies control and peace. It's just a question of patience and faith.

6 You can't use other actives with retinoids

Incorrect. Retinoids work really well if partnered with synergistic actives, such as azelaic acid and niacinamide, for conditions such as acne and pigmentation. What is key is to ensure barrier health is preserved, first and foremost. Stronger actives, for example benzoyl peroxide and vitamin C, may need timing strategies or alternate-day use to give your skin a breather and ensure tolerance. In sensitive skin, introduce one active at a time, ensuring tolerance is achieved with each step in isolation before adding in the next.

7 Using a retinoid once or twice a week works just as well

You will achieve best results when you use a retinoid daily. Therefore, if you find that you're still skipping a couple of days a week on a regular basis, after a decent trial period of six weeks or more, you should lower the intensity of yours.

8 You can't use retinoids when breastfeeding

This is incorrect. Retinoids are not used in pregnancy because vitamin A is a signalling molecule in the developing foetus, so it's advised that expecting mums avoid any excess. But after the baby is born, it's fine to use a topical retinoid on your face. Just avoid any direct transference from your skin onto your baby's skin, to avoid irritation.

RETINIZATION:
WHAT TO EXPECT AND HOW TO HANDLE IT

Starting a retinoid is a bit like beginning a new workout – your skin might ache in new ways as it adjusts to this powerful influence. Expect a little flaking (especially around the mouth and chin), tightness, sensitivity, and possibly a breakout or two (that's purging, see above).

To ease the transition, go in gently. Start with a lower-strength, non-prescription retinoid, and buffer it with moisturizer (see Chapter 6, page 126). Apply on alternate nights at first; daily use can come later. There's no rush, and trust me, consistency trumps intensity.

Retinoid dermatitis – red, sore, irritated skin – usually results from going too strong, too fast, too often, or from layering on too many actives at once. I always tell patients to focus on building tolerance first through increasing frequency. Only then do we reassess the strength of your retinoid, typically every three months.

Deciding if you need to increase the strength of your retinoid then becomes easy, once your skin is tolerant to your current one. If you've reached your goals, there's no need to go further – keep going with what you're using. If your skin is tolerant but you've not yet reached your goals – go ahead and increase the strength.

NOTES FROM THE CLINIC

I encourage patients to view this transition period as something exciting – your skin is changing! It's exactly what we want. You didn't arrive here overnight and resetting your skin's behaviour takes a little time, as all good things do, so stay the course.

The bottom line:
Stay the course. Retinization is temporary – and the glow once you're through it is worth it.

2 AZELAIC ACID

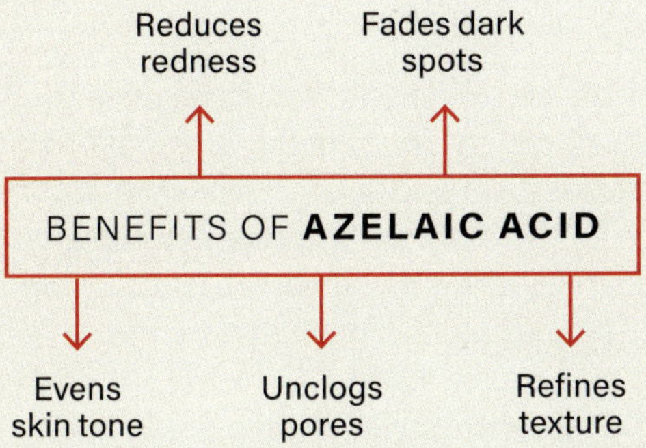

This is one of the most underrated multitaskers in the skincare world. I feel I have been championing this active since the beginning of my social media career (so about a decade!). It's rarely the ingredient people get excited about (assuming they've heard of it in the first place). It doesn't generate headlines like retinoids or spark controversy like acids. But, in truth, I couldn't operate a successful clinic without it.

Endlessly versatile and surprisingly well tolerated, azelaic acid has an impressive CV and a place in nearly every skin routine I build.

Crucially, if your skin can't tolerate a retinoid (yet), azelaic acid might just be the gateway ingredient that makes it possible.

WHAT IS IT?

Azelaic acid is a naturally occurring dicarboxylic acid, originally derived from grains, although these days it's synthetically produced for stability and purity. It is available over the counter in concentrations from 5–10%, and on prescription at 15–20%.

It's one of the few actives that works well, whatever I'm treating. Much like a retinoid, it works *inside* the cells, acting at multiple checkpoints. It's as useful in treating acne as it is in tackling pigmentation; it even has anti-inflammatory and antioxidant powers. It's a balance that's rare in actives; an ingredient that's both calming, coaching sensitive skin to settle down, yet profoundly transformative.

HOW IT WORKS

Azelaic acid does *a lot*. It inhibits tyrosinase, the enzyme responsible for melanin production, which helps fade pigmentation. It's especially well suited to treat post-inflammatory marks from acne because of its other helpful properties.

Azelaic acid prevents breakouts by normalizing keratinization, so it stops sticky skin cells clumping up and clogging your pores. And it helps destroy *C. acnes*, the acne-triggering bacteria (so no need for topical antibiotics and the risk of antibacterial resistance).

It calms redness and inflammation, making it ideal for tackling everything from rosacea to acne and even perioral dermatitis. The only thing it doesn't do is support collagen production, but when combined with niacinamide or a retinoid, this isn't a concern.

It's one of the few actives that plays nicely with skin in turmoil. I find that when I use azelaic acid, it turns the dial down on irritability and increases tolerance to whatever ingredient I try adding in later. For example, someone with fiery rosacea treated with azelaic acid for 6 months might well find their skin now accepts a retinoid, where it wouldn't have before.

WHAT IT TREATS

Azelaic acid is incredibly versatile and, crucially for anyone stopping a retinoid when they start planning to conceive, is pregnancy-safe and an excellent alternative in many instances. It's well suited to treating:

- **Acne** (both the inflammatory and comedonal types)
- **Pigmentation** (including post-blemish marks and melasma)
- **Rosacea** (especially papulopustular type)
- **Perioral dermatitis**

HOW FAST YOU'LL SEE RESULTS

You might notice a calming effect within a couple of weeks; redness fades, bumps flatten, and skin is less reactive. Pigmentation and clogged pores take a little longer: expect to see changes over 8–12 weeks with consistent use. Its benefits build over time, and the longer you stick with it, the better your skin will behave.

COMMON AZELAIC ACID MYTHS

Azelaic acid is relatively myth-free compared to our friends, the retinoids. But here are a couple I hear quite frequently in the clinic.

1 Azelaic acid is too gentle to do much

This is actually something I heard anecdotally during my dermatology training. But just because it's well tolerated that doesn't mean it's ineffective. There is good evidence for its use in all the aforementioned inflammatory skin disorders. What's more, compliance is high. This is incredibly important when you want people to stick with a routine for months and beyond.

2 You don't need azelaic acid if you're already using a retinoid

Actually, the two pair beautifully. Azelaic acid enhances any results you might achieve with a retinoid in both acne and pigmentation. I often prescribe them together, using azelaic acid in the morning and a retinoid at night. It also adds an anti-inflammatory edge that helps with retinoid tolerance if started beforehand and it helps keep a lid on purging.

WHAT TO EXPECT AND HOW TO USE IT

Azelaic acid doesn't usually have a 'drama phase' like retinoids – no flaking, no purging, no major barrier disruptions. That said, some people experience mild stinging, dryness, or a bit of itchiness at first. That's all normal and tends to settle within a week or two.

My advice? Start with alternate-day use, and use buffering if you're nervous (see page 126), applying it *after* moisturizer. Once your skin's comfortable, you can move it closer to the skin. It's very forgiving, so it's often the first active I introduce in routines for sensitive, redness-prone or hyperpigmented skin. And yes, it plays beautifully with other actives.

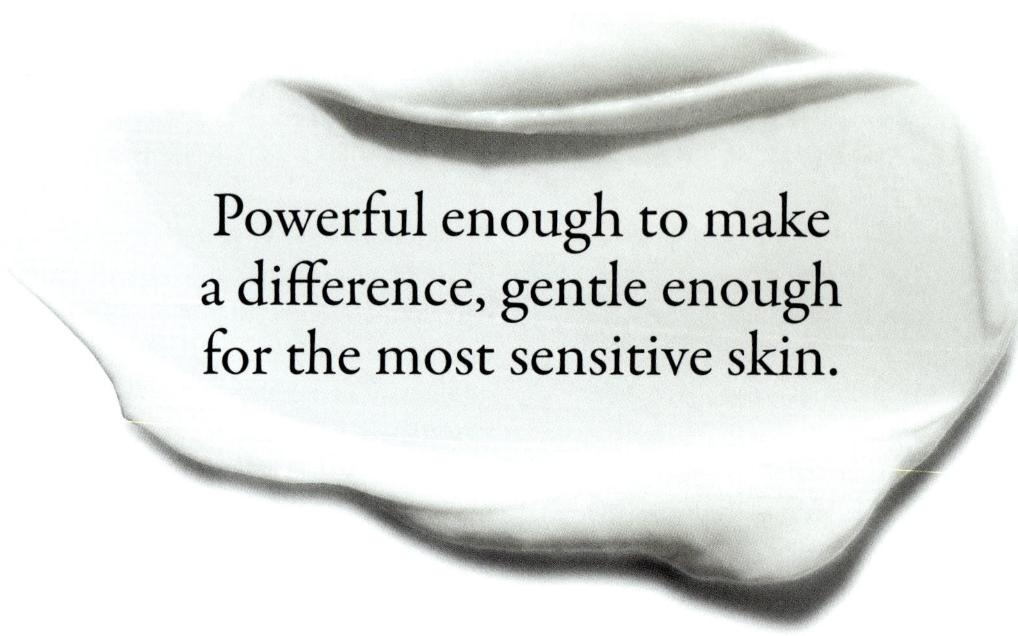

WHO AZELAIC ACID IS BEST FOR

Honestly, almost everyone – it's powerful enough to make a big difference to skin quality, yet gentle enough for the most sensitive skin. It's also a dream for anyone who has more than one skin issue, like melasma *and* rosacea. And it's the ingredient I often reach for first when treating my pregnant and lactating patients.

WHEN TO AVOID IT

If your skin is already over-exfoliated or sensitized from actives, pause all of them, repair your skin barrier, then introduce it gently.

The bottom line:
Azelaic acid is the quiet overachiever in your skincare routine. If you want bright, clear and resilient skin with minimal drama, it's for you.

3 NIACINAMIDE

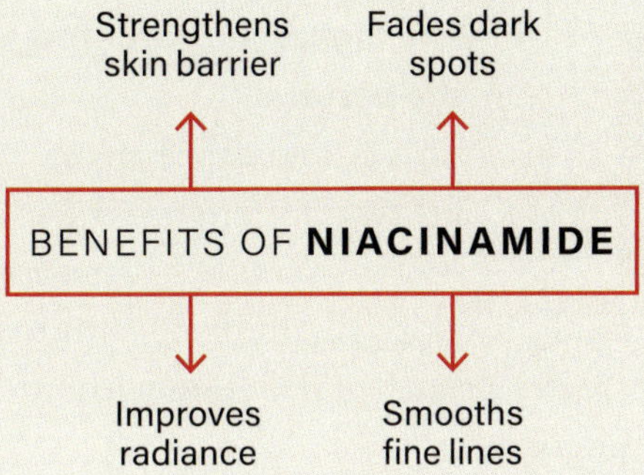

Now, let's talk about the ultimate crowd-pleaser: niacinamide. Niacinamide has become a staple in modern skincare, offering a dizzying array of benefits while being very well tolerated. It's affordable, adaptable and makes a smart addition to almost any routine.

That said, its popularity has led to a bit of confusion when it comes to strength – more is not always better. And just because it's everywhere, that doesn't mean it should be used indiscriminately.

Think of niacinamide as your skin's personal trainer: it strengthens, soothes and boosts performance over time. Similar to azelaic acid, it's a balanced ingredient with both corrective and calming benefits. It helps everything else work better.

WHAT IS IT?

Niacinamide, also known as vitamin B3, is a water-soluble vitamin found naturally in our food and widely used in skincare for its impressive multitasking capabilities. It typically comes in concentrations anywhere between 2% and 20%.

HOW IT WORKS

Niacinamide works inside skin cells to restore and optimize skin function. It boosts ceramide production, improving the strength of your skin barrier. It brightens and makes skin more even-toned by inhibiting melanosome transfer, so that fewer parcels of melanin get delivered into your keratinocytes. It soothes inflammation, making it a great support act for conditions such as acne and rosacea. Finally, it provides antioxidant protection against environmental stressors and helps preserve fibroblast energy production, by maintaining healthy mitochondria. Indirectly, this helps support collagen production. It's a generalist rather than a specialist. But a very good one.

WHAT IT TREATS

Niacinamide is helpful if enlarged, clogged-up pores and uneven texture are on your agenda of problems to solve. It's useful in both acne and rosacea, helping to calm inflamed blemishes, making strong actives easier to tolerate. It's also something I add to almost every routine for photo-aged skin to restore vibrancy.

HOW FAST YOU'LL SEE RESULTS

Expect to see improvements in hydration and skin smoothness within 2–4 weeks. Visible changes in fine lines and pigmentation take a little longer, so give it 8–12 weeks to see results.

Consistency is key. As it's generally non-irritating, this is one of the easier actives to use daily (and long-term).

COMMON NIACINAMIDE MYTHS

1

The higher the percentage, the better

This is one of the biggest misconceptions out there. More isn't more when it comes to niacinamide. Pushing past 10% increases the risk of irritation without better outcomes.

2

It can't be used with vitamin C

This is outdated advice. Modern niacinamide preparations are stable and play nicely with almost all actives, including vitamin C. Just don't pile everything on at once. Retinoids and niacinamide are especially good together, as the ceramide-boosting ability of niacinamide helps to minimize retinoid-related irritation.

3

It should be used as a stand-alone step

I think not. Niacinamide is a good-natured active that can happily be combined with others in a single formula for efficiency. Let's not waste time on more steps in our routine than we need.

WHAT TO EXPECT AND HOW TO USE IT

Introducing niacinamide is generally smooth sailing. You'll rarely encounter the irritation or purging you might associate with retinoids, for example. However, when used at very high concentrations, it can occasionally cause redness or tingling, especially in sensitive skin. Start low and build up your strength over time.

WHO NIACINAMIDE IS BEST FOR

Niacinamide is a true all-rounder. It's as helpful for those with oily or acne-prone skin as it is for sensitive or redness-prone complexions, thanks to its calming, anti-inflammatory properties.

If you're struggling with barrier repair or dehydration, niacinamide supports the skin's natural defences and restores balance. And for actives newcomers, it's one of the easiest ingredients to start with. It helps build skin tolerance, which will make introducing other actives easier while still delivering visible benefits.

WHEN TO AVOID IT

If your product contains 10% niacinamide (or higher) and you're seeing signs of irritation, have a break and scale the strength back.

The bottom line:
I rely on niacinamide a lot. It improves resilience, regulates function and smooths the path for more targeted actives. And when used appropriately, it's the kind of ingredient that makes your whole routine work better. Think of it as skincare's equivalent of a good night's sleep.

4 SALICYLIC ACID

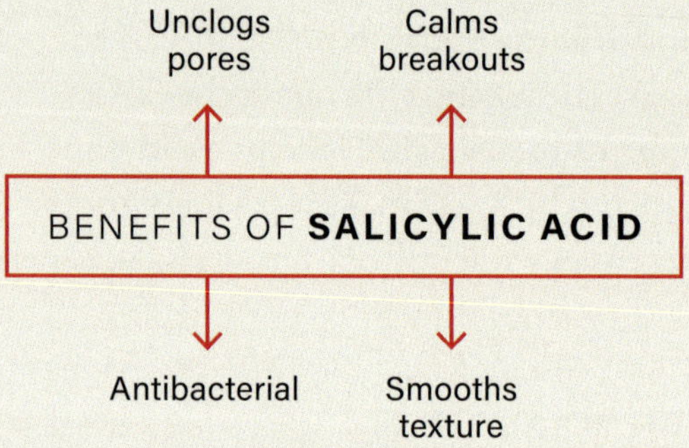

This is perhaps my favourite of the true acids. Its ability to penetrate deeply into the oily environment of our pores makes it one I reach for time and again, whether it's to tackle breakouts or textured skin, or just to cut through the shine of an oily T-zone.

WHAT IS IT?

Salicylic acid is a beta hydroxy acid (BHA) that comes from willow bark and is from the same family as aspirin. The beauty of salicylic acid is that it's oil-soluble, so it can get to places that its water-soluble cousins, the alpha hydroxy acids (AHAs), just can't reach.

You'll find it in skincare products at a strength of 0.5% to 2%. There are all manner of preparations containing BHAs, but again, I prefer a leave-on product that you can carefully dose, rather than a BHA cleanser or toner, where you are unsure where and how much is actually being deposited on the skin.

HOW IT WORKS

Salicylic acid dissolves the glue that binds skin cells and sebum together. This loosens any clogs or debris (known as sebaceous filaments), and helps clear congestion in your pores, to eliminate open and closed comedones. The result is smooth, clear and predictable skin.

It will also exfoliate the surface of your skin, improving texture and reducing the appearance of any dark marks that previous blemishes have left behind.

It's powerfully anti-inflammatory, meaning that it will lessen the redness and swelling of your blemishes, so they disappear more speedily. This is further compounded by its antibacterial and antifungal properties.

WHAT IT TREATS

Its combination of attributes means it's an absolute hero when it comes to tackling breakouts at multiple stages in their evolution. It can also help treat body issues such as ingrown hairs, folliculitis and keratosis pilaris (see Chapter 8, pages 157–71).

HOW FAST YOU'LL SEE RESULTS

Exfoliants work quite fast, so you can expect to see smoother skin within a few days and the redness in blemishes might well be better in a similar timeframe. Clearing out pores takes longer, so allow at least 6 weeks for improvement.

Likewise, improving post-inflammatory marks takes a couple of skin cycles, so give it 6–12 weeks.

COMMON SALICYLIC ACID MYTHS

1

Salicylic acid is too harsh for sensitive skin
I hear this a lot. In my experience, it's often what surrounds salicylic acid in the formula, rather than the salicylic acid per se. It's common for salicylic acid to be paired with denatured alcohol, as it makes it penetrate skin quickly and absorb speedily. This is desirable if you have oily skin, but less so for those with sensitivity, where it can leave skin dry, irritable and tight. Formulas with salicylic acid that skip denatured alcohol and utilize barrier-supporting ingredients like squalane are usually fine for sensitive skin.

2

It's only for teens
While teens do benefit from salicylic acid to tackle oily skin and breakouts, there are plenty of upsides in terms of texture improvement and general clarity for adults, provided it's formulated with care.

3

It's unsafe for pregnancy
While we do recommend avoiding oral salicylic acid (aspirin) in pregnancy, when used topically in small amounts on facial skin, salicylic acid is safe up to 2% strength.

WHAT TO EXPECT AND HOW TO USE IT

We aren't changing what happens inside the cells with salicylic acid – it works on the outside. That means you can use it episodically, such as for a one-off blemish. Or you can use it every day to help keep pores clear. Adapt its use to your needs. Just take care when it comes to combining it with other products, unless it has been intentionally co-formulated with synergistic actives.

I tend to avoid using salicylic acid at the same time as retinoids (separate them and use your BHA in the morning). I also don't recommend layering with vitamin C, as it tends to be too irritating.

WHO SALICYLIC ACID IS BEST FOR

Salicylic acid is best for tackling acne, particularly where skin is oily, congested and prone to visible pores. Its exfoliating action makes it a go-to for body issues, as we'll see in Chapter 8 (see pages 157–71).

WHEN TO AVOID IT

If you're allergic to aspirin, steer clear of salicylic acid – try azelaic acid instead.

The bottom line:
Salicylic acid is a brilliant addition to a routine for acne-prone teens and adults alike, when you want to harness its ability to clear and calm pores from the inside-out in your trouble zones.

5 BENZOYL PEROXIDE

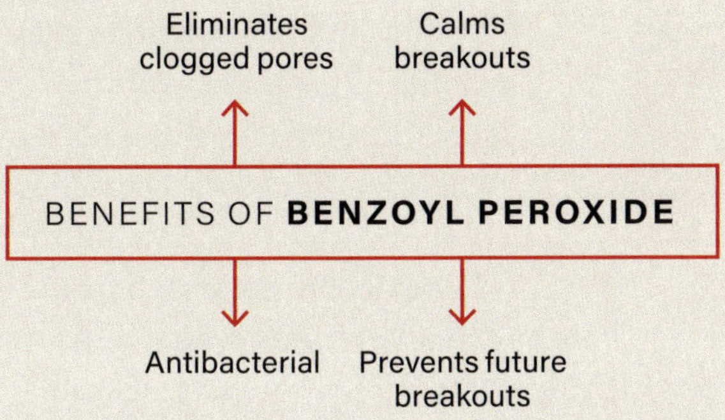

When angry red blemishes need fast resolution, this is the ingredient I reach for first. It may not have the allure of a retinoid or the multitasking charm of azelaic acid, but benzoyl peroxide has stood the test of time, and for good reason. It is direct, no-nonsense and highly effective.

WHAT IS IT?

Benzoyl peroxide (BPO) is an organic peroxide and a potent oxidizing agent used primarily to treat acne. It's available over the counter in the UK, typically at 5% strength, and it's also available in prescription in a variety of helpful combinations. It works topically and, unlike many other acne treatments, it doesn't lead to bacterial resistance. That's one of the reasons it's so useful – it's a workhorse that never tires.

HOW IT WORKS

Benzoyl peroxide delivers a three-pronged attack against breakouts. When it is applied to the skin, reactive oxygen species (ROS) are released which kill the bacteria *C. acnes*, a critical player in acne. It's also anti-inflammatory, calming the redness and swelling that make blemishes feel sore and look angry. Finally, it helps tackle comedones, those little timebombs lying in wait to explode into inflamed spots.

WHAT IT TREATS

Benzoyl peroxide is particularly effective against inflammatory acne, both papules and pustules, and it can help curb early-stage cystic spots before they progress. It also works to clear clogged pores.

I tend to reach for BPO when someone is struggling with fast-evolving breakouts and needs visible change quickly, especially during hormonal flare-ups or in teenage skin.

HOW FAST YOU'LL SEE RESULTS

Most patients notice a reduction in spot size and redness within just a few days. Its fast onset is one of the reasons I love it for a pre-event rescue or for a bride-to-be feeling the pressure. With consistent use, you'll see fewer new blemishes and faster healing within a couple of weeks.

COMMON BENZOYL PEROXIDE MYTHS

1

It's too harsh for sensitive skin
While BPO undoubtedly has irritation potential, like salicylic acid, a lot depends on the vehicle of the treatment you're using to deliver it onto the skin. Some BPO gels are loaded with alcohol, which helps it penetrate deep into the pore (useful), but can strip the skin barrier (not ideal). More modern formulas balance actives with hydrating occlusive ingredients, such as silicones. In practice, I find that tolerability can be increased by sparing use on targeted areas *over* your moisturizer rather than underneath it.

2

Stronger is better
Not necessarily. I typically recommend 2.5–5% BPO – this is the sweet spot. A higher strength increases the likelihood of irritation without dramatically improving efficacy.

3

It can't be used with retinoids
It *can*, but timing matters. BPO can damage the delicate retinoid structure, rendering them ineffective, so I recommend using BPO in the morning and your retinoid at night (unless you're using a prescription combination product).

SMART PRESCRIPTION COMBINATIONS

Tackling acne at multiple checkpoints is a proven strategy for results and the pharmaceutical industry has made it easier than ever by combining BPO with other synergistic ingredients in a single formula. It also makes sticking with a routine that bit easier, as fewer steps are needed.

BPO + retinoid (Epiduo): to clear pores and reduce inflammation. I use this when someone struggles with committing to more than a once-daily regime.

BPO + antibiotic (Duac): to boost the bacteria-fighting properties even further and reduce resistance risk to the antibiotic. I particularly like the vehicle Duac is formulated with, as it's really hydrating, helping to offset the drying effect of BPO.

WHO BENZOYL PEROXIDE IS BEST FOR

Benzoyl peroxide is best for teens and adults dealing with inflamed acne, especially when blemishes are red, tender and in need of rapid resolution. It's also pregnancy-safe.This active is an important option for those people who have previously relied on topical antibiotics alone that no longer deliver results, due to bacterial resistance.

WHEN TO AVOID IT

- If you're allergic to benzoyl peroxide (patch test first! – see box, page 151).
- If your skin is barrier-compromised or currently over-exfoliated.
- If you're worried about bleaching towels or pillowcases; it's a real thing – use white ones.
- Don't use it at the same time as hydroquinone, an ingredient we use to fade hyperpigmentation (it can temporarily stain the skin).

The bottom line:
Benzoyl peroxide is the bazooka in your acne arsenal. It's powerful when used with care. It won't give you the skin-enhancing benefits of a retinoid or azelaic acid, but when spots are flaring, few things rival its speed and reliability.

6 VITAMIN C

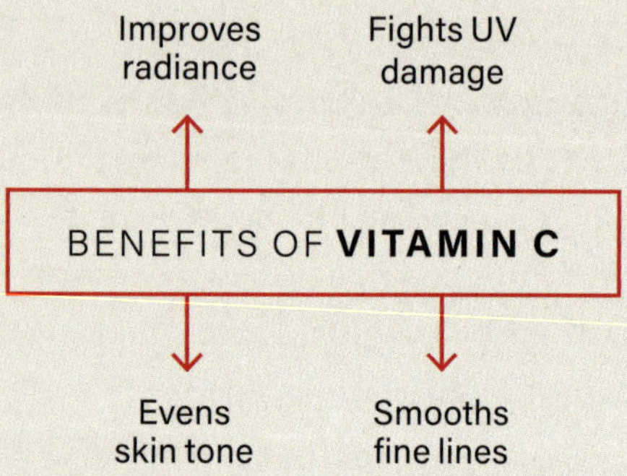

If there was a skincare popularity contest, vitamin C would be a hot contender for the top spot. It's adored for its radiance-boosting properties and is one of the fundamental actives when it comes to achieving an even-toned, healthy complexion.

WHAT IS IT?

Vitamin C, or ascorbic acid, is a powerful antioxidant that our bodies need but can't manufacture, so we have to import it, either through our diet or through our skincare. In the skin, it plays a critical role in collagen production, pigmentation regulation and environmental defence.

The gold-standard form of vitamin C used in clinical research is L-ascorbic acid – it's the most biologically active and one of the most common forms found in skincare products. But it comes with a catch: L-ascorbic acid is notoriously unstable and can oxidize in light, heat and air, rendering it ineffective. It's also water-soluble and struggles to penetrate the skin's barrier, which is rich in oils (and as we know, oil and water don't mix).

To improve absorption, formulas are typically adjusted to a pH of around 3.5, where more of the vitamin C exists in an uncharged form that can slip into the skin more easily. However, this acidity can be a double-edged sword – while the skin naturally prefers a slightly acidic environment, very low pH levels can be irritating, especially for sensitive skin.

HOW IT WORKS

Vitamin C in your routine works hard. It boosts collagen production by acting as a cofactor for the enzymes involved in its assembly into strong fibres. It is powerfully preventative when it comes to the signs of ageing, because it protects skin from oxidative stress by neutralizing ROS from UV light and pollution before they can cause damage inside our skin cells. It also inhibits tyrosinase, the pivotal enzyme that drives melanin production, helping to fade hyperpigmentation and brighten the skin. Finally, it supports healthy wound healing.

When you add this all up, it translates to vibrant, firm, more even-toned skin that holds its structure better as you age.

WHAT IT TREATS

Vitamin C is ideal for treating uneven tone and pigmentation while reviving skin that looks dull or lacking radiance. I add it to routines for patients tackling concerns such as premature ageing and melasma.

Vitamin C is also a foundational active in any skin longevity strategy to complement the use of daily sunscreen. It is especially important for women entering perimenopause and menopause, where collagen loss accelerates dramatically in the first few years.

It's also the first active I'll introduce when building a routine for someone in their twenties whose skin is in good shape and whose goal is simply optimized maintenance.

If there was a skincare popularity contest, vitamin C would be a hot contender for the top spot.

HOW FAST YOU'LL SEE RESULTS

You'll start to see a noticeable glow and increased clarity in 2–4 weeks. Improvement in fine lines takes longer to see – think 3–6 months of consistent use. As with retinoids, the benefits accumulate over time.

COMMON VITAMIN C MYTHS

1

All vitamin C serums are the same
Not at all. Formulation is everything – stability, concentration and their delivery system all affect how well a vitamin C product gets into the skin.

2

Stronger is better
Nope. Higher concentrations (20%+) can cause more irritation, especially in sensitive skin, with no additional benefit. A strength of 10–15% is usually the sweet spot.

3

Vitamin C can't be used with other actives
Incorrect. It plays beautifully with most actives we use to combat the signs of ageing, including both retinoids and niacinamide. In fact, combining vitamin C with the antioxidants ferulic acid and vitamin E in a formula strengthens defences even further, improving product stability and delivering more reliable protection against daily oxidative stress.

4

Vitamin C causes purging
It doesn't affect the way pores function, so vitamin C has no role in treating acne (this often surprises people), nor should it trigger purging. If you find you're breaking out with vitamin C, it's likely due to irritation, or it's due to something else in the formula clogging your pores. Take a break and try switching to a more gentle vitamin C product.

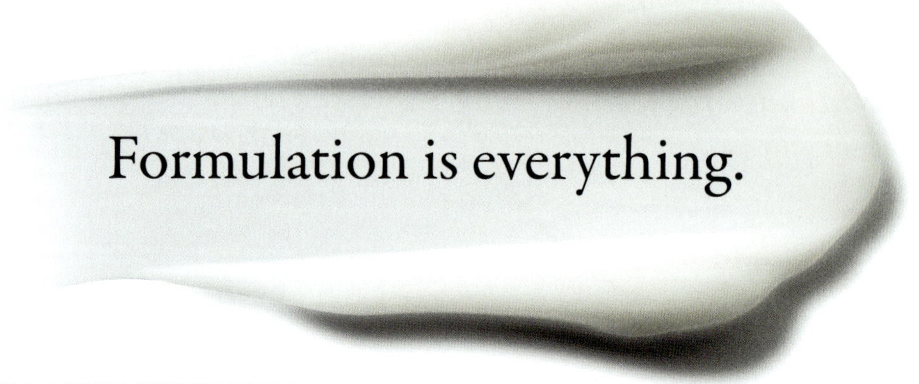

WHAT ARE VITAMIN C DERIVATIVES?

While we know a lot about L-ascorbic acid and how it affects the skin, it is not necessarily the easiest ingredient to use and I've seen a lot of patients struggle with it over the years. I've also struggled to use it myself – my redness-prone skin simply finds it too irritating.

This is where vitamin C derivatives come in. By using chemical 'add-ons' that are stuck onto the L-ascorbic acid molecule, we render it more stable and better able to penetrate the skin near to its natural pH, thus avoiding unnecessary irritation.

Vitamin C derivatives include:

- THD Ascorbate (Tetrahexyldecyl Ascorbate): add-on of fatty acid chains, delivering an oil-soluble molecule which is good for brightening in dry skin.
- Ascorbyl Glucoside: add-on of a sugar molecule, which enhances stability and makes it suitable for sensitive skin.
- Magnesium Ascorbyl Phosphate (MAP): add-on of phosphate groups, which increases stability and reduces acidity, making it less irritating.

These derivatives are better tolerated, making them a great option for barrier-compromised or rosacea-prone skin.

There is a caveat. We have less clinical data on many of these compared to L-ascorbic acid, so while they're promising, they're not all equally proven. This is an area where research is evolving and nuance matters. However, from a practical standpoint, their increased stability and tolerability can make them far better suited for life on your bathroom shelf.

PACKAGING AND STORAGE

There is nothing more annoying than discovering that you've left your expensive bottle of vitamin C serum unscrewed and exposure to the air has turned it orange or brown. It happens to us all at some point.

Fortunately, clever packaging innovation can help solve vitamin C's inherent instability issue. Look for anything that's opaque and airless. Anhydrous (water-free) formulas are also a smart idea as these are more stable. Finally, keep your vitamin C somewhere that reduces the risk of product breakdown with minimal exposure to heat and light – ideally in its box, somewhere cool.

HOW TO USE IT

Vitamin C should always be used in the morning in order to fortify your skin's defences against the environment, alongside your sunscreen. Apply it directly after cleansing to maximize absorption.

WHO VITAMIN C IS BEST FOR

Vitamin C is best for anyone concerned with dullness, uneven tone or the first signs of ageing. It's a smart choice for those looking to take a preventative approach to collagen loss, and it's particularly valuable if you're prone to pigmentation. For perimenopausal and menopausal skin, where collagen preservation becomes critical, it's a must.

WHEN TO AVOID IT

If your skin is actively breaking out, there are better-suited ingredients when it comes to tackling post-acne pigmentation. I see a lot of people using vitamin C incorrectly in this way. I do, however, bring it into a routine once breakouts are stabilized and we refocus on healthy ageing.

If breakouts flare, I recommend pressing pause on vitamin C and prioritizing anti-blemish ingredients such as salicylic acid, benzoyl peroxide and azelaic acid first. It's worth mentioning that it should never be combined with BPO – it will inactivate your vitamin C.

The bottom line:

Vitamin C is one of the few ingredients with good clinical data and a clear biological role in building healthy collagen, providing antioxidant protection and supporting pigmentation control. When used correctly, over time, it will help deliver bright, clear and more resilient skin.

MATCHMAKING YOUR ACTIVES AND CONCERN

Clever combinations add up to more than the sum of their parts. Here's how you use chemistry to multitask.

STEP	RETINOIDS	AZELAIC ACID	NIACINAMIDE	SALICYLIC ACID	BENZOYL PEROXIDE	VITAMIN C
Acne	✓	✓	✓	✓	✓	
Clogged pores	✓	✓	✓	✓	✓	
Hyperpigmentation	✓	✓	✓			✓
Redness/ Rosacea		✓	✓			
Fine lines/ Wrinkles	✓		✓			✓
Uneven texture	✓	✓	✓	✓		✓

These rules aren't hard and fast: you can often use retinoids in rosacea once it's under control, for instance.

Remember there's no need to use all the actives ticked per concern at once; it's important to build your routine carefully, one or two actives at a time.

Head to the next chapter where I put this all together for you.

OTHER ACTIVES: HONOURABLE MENTIONS

While still valuable, these ingredients may have limited evidence or are indicated in more specific scenarios.

BAKUCHIOL

Bakuchiol is a smart plant extract that behaves like a retinoid, but isn't one. It is often dismissed as a kind of poor man's retinol, but this underestimates its capabilities. Bakuchiol helps to reduce fine lines, pigmentation and breakouts, all with a gentle hand. It's especially useful in sensitive or blemish-prone skin, and it shines in pregnancy when traditional retinoids are off the table. It's also an effective antioxidant and is suitable for use during the day, unlike retinoids. Finally, it has an emerging role in skin longevity (see Chapter 9, page 174) that makes it complementary to a healthy ageing skin strategy.[vi]

LACTIC ACID

Lactic acid stands apart as the rare exfoliant that refines and replenishes in equal measure. Unlike harsher alpha hydroxy acids (AHAs), it smooths skin gently while boosting hydration, thanks to its role as a natural humectant and a key component of the skin's innate moisturizing system. Its larger molecular size means it penetrates more slowly, reducing irritation, while also helping to stimulate ceramide production and strengthen the skin barrier. Useful, especially in those with dry skin who crave more radiance.

HYDROQUINONE

Hydroquinone is the gold standard for fading stubborn pigmentation for good reason. It works by directly interfering with melanin production at the source, switching off overactive pigment cells with precision by inhibiting tyrosinase. Unlike cosmetic brighteners that can take time to act, hydroquinone is decisive and fast-acting, making it my mainstay for tackling melasma, but also for tackling stubborn sun spots and post-acne marks, when gentler options don't deliver the desired outcome.

But with that potency comes the need for care: it's a short-term solution best used in well-structured pulsed cycles, in rotation with other non-prescription tyrosinase inhibitors and under expert guidance. This is critical. In the UK, it's only available on prescription and is most helpful at a strength of 4%. In the right hands, hydroquinone is a powerful reset button for uneven skin tone.

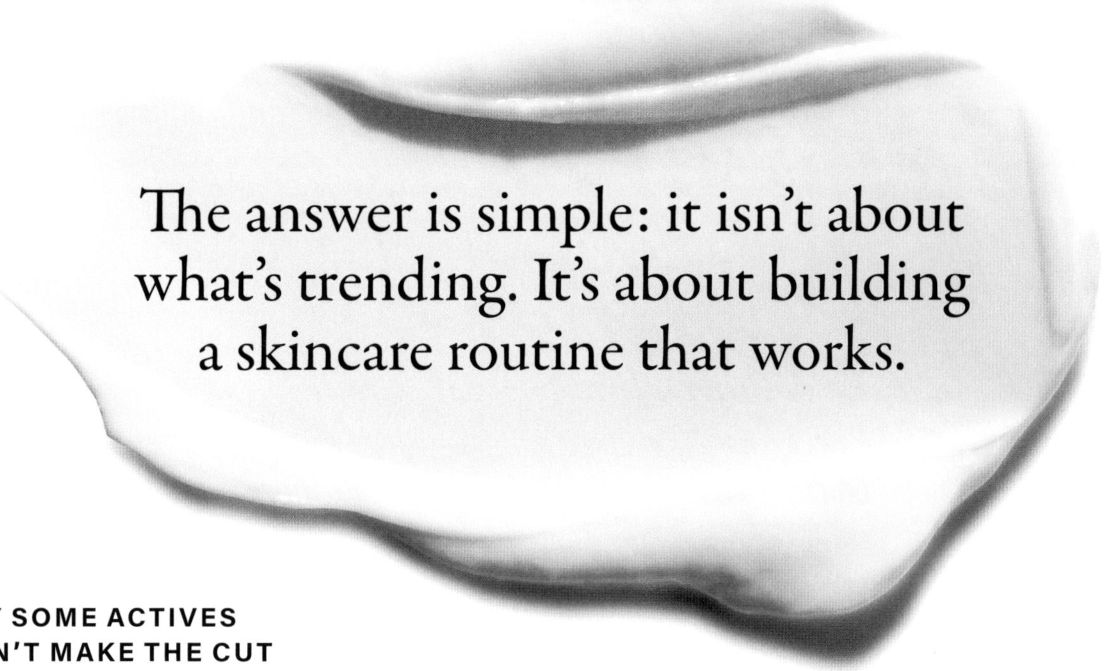

The answer is simple: it isn't about what's trending. It's about building a skincare routine that works.

WHY SOME ACTIVES DIDN'T MAKE THE CUT

You might be wondering why certain buzzy ingredients aren't featured in this chapter. Where's glycolic acid, for instance, or peptides, or snail mucin? The answer is simple: it isn't about what's trending. It's about what works and has continued to work over the course of years in my practice.

I've deliberately focused on the actives that have consistently delivered meaningful, measurable changes for my patients over time. These are ingredients I trust to form the backbone of a targeted skincare routine, ones I can combine safely and effectively without triggering confusion or irritation. That doesn't mean every other ingredient is 'bad' – it just means they're not in my core toolkit.

Take glycolic acid. It's a powerful exfoliant, but in practice I find it too aggressive relative to the impact it delivers, especially when paired with other actives that yield bigger bang for your buck, such as retinoids. That's why I prefer gentler AHAs, such as lactic acid, which are more forgiving for sensitive or reactive skin.

Then there are peptides. While they sound promising (and are often marketed with great enthusiasm), they don't yet have the independent clinical evidence to justify a starring role. They may well be helpful, but I'd rather build a routine around proven heavy-hitters than hypothetical ones. In an efficient routine, where you want the maximum impact in the fewest steps, you must prioritize.

As for novelty ingredients like snail mucin or bee venom – they might have social media traction, but they're not grounded in science yet. I prioritize ingredients with a clear mechanism of action, reliable studies and long-term, real-world results.

So, if you're scanning this chapter looking for what's hot on TikTok and not finding it – that's exactly the point. This isn't about hype. It's about building a skincare routine that works.

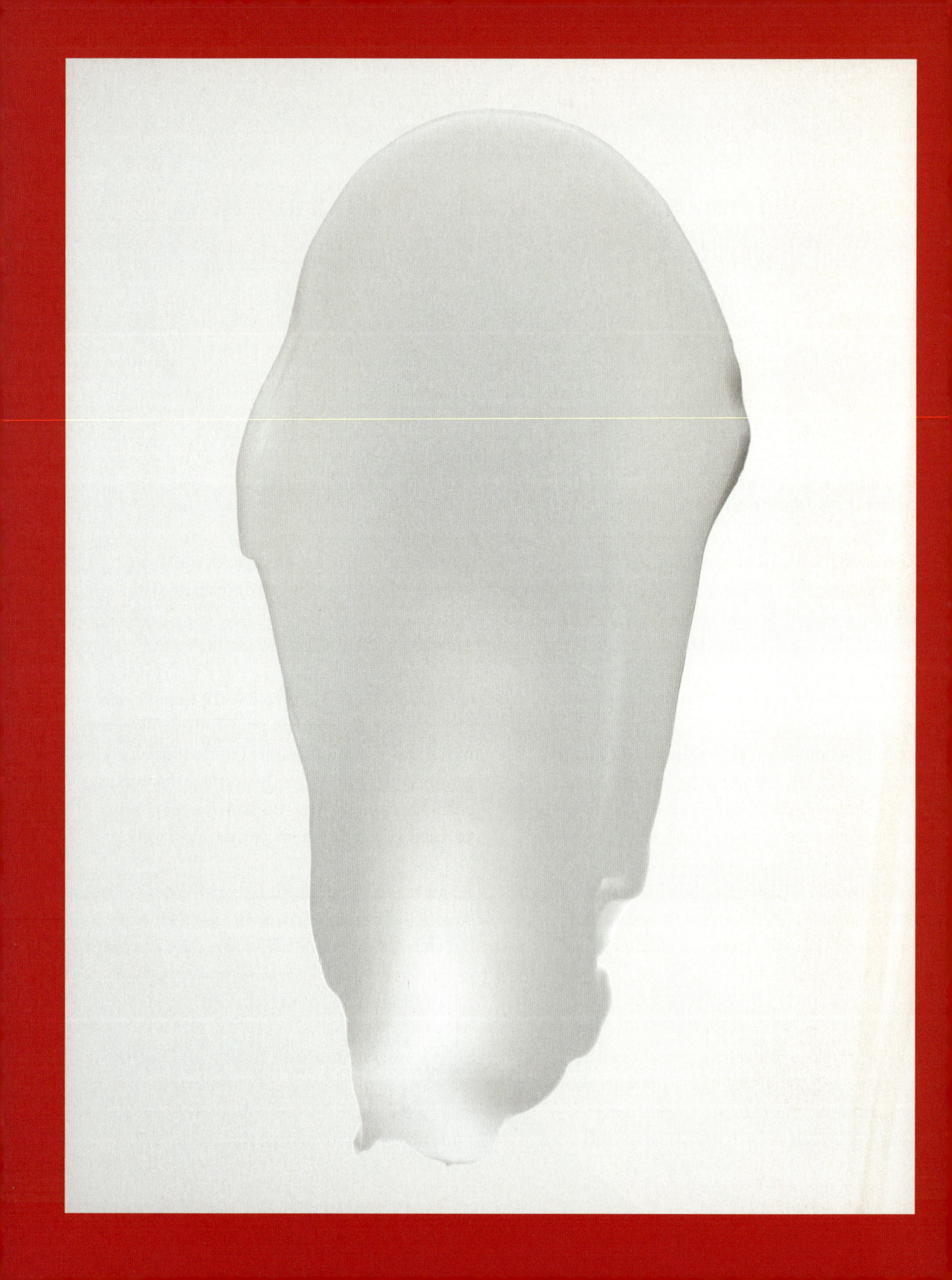

6

Building a Skincare Routine

THE FOUR PILLARS IN ACTION

When building a skincare routine, we want the minimum number of steps to deliver the maximum impact. So, let's drill down into The Four Pillars (see page 76).

1 CLEANSE

Despite the endless choice, cleansing does not need to be complicated and should do no harm. For most people, a gentle rinse-off, non-foaming gel cleanser is the best tool for the job. Every form of cleansing disrupts the skin barrier – even water alone – so the aim is simply to minimize that disruption by avoiding unnecessary irritants such as fragrance, foaming agents and heavy oil or balm textures that might clog pores. A simple wash-off gel cleanser suits the majority of us, given the prevalence of sensitivity and combination skin.

Conscious cleansing is key. While we often perform our cleanse on automatic pilot, with a bit of thought it can be done effectively without doing harm. This sets the perfect tone for the rest of your routine.

Cleansing is a functional step: its role is to remove what does not belong on the skin, not to treat conditions such as acne, rosacea or pigmentation, and when it's done gently, it lays the foundation for everything that follows.

REMOVING MAKE-UP

Feel free to use a dedicated eye make-up remover to deal with stubborn mascara and eyeliner before your cleanse to minimize the need for friction. Cleansing afterwards ensures that any residue that migrates from the eye area onto the cheeks is thoroughly removed.

HOW TO USE A RINSE-OFF GEL CLEANSER

1. Make sure your face and neck are clear of anything that would impede you from being able to cleanse thoroughly. That may involve taking off jewellery, tying your hair up or using a headband to get it away from your face. You might even want to try towelling wrist bands to minimize water dripping down your sleeves.

2. Wet your skin first. Water temperature is key. Not too hot, not too cold – tepid is best.

3. Take the right amount of product. Use a 10-pence-sized amount (about 2.5cm/ 1 inch in diameter) in the morning and double the amount at night, when there's more to remove from your skin.

4. Use your fingertips to massage your cleanser into the skin. If you must use something to lift the cleanser off, opt for a very fine-textured, wet muslin cloth or wet cotton pads. Remember the aim is to remove *just* the cleanser, so resist the urge to exert force and exfoliate! I find that almost everything can be removed with a 60-second fingertip cleanse. Set a timer on your phone, it's longer than you think. Use the time to breathe with a long, calming exhale. Close your eyes and take a moment to connect with yourself. Allow cleansing to become a mini meditation.

5. Rinse clear with tepid water, ensuring you remove all traces of cleanser. It is not uncommon to miss areas like the temples or hairline, so rinse thoroughly and systematically. Cleansing in the shower makes rinsing easy, so feel free to do this (just turn the temperature to tepid).

6. Gently pat your face dry with a clean towel. It can be tempting to be rough when drying, but think of your skin as precious silk and handle it with care.

2 ACTIVATE

After the last chapter, you should now be an actives pro. Let's put what you've learned into motion.

Actives are best applied to clean skin in order for them to be thoroughly absorbed, hence why they are the next step after cleansing. If an ingredient is to have an impact, it must get to its desired destination within the skin. Our skin is very good at keeping things out, which is why we generally want an unobstructed path for our actives.

The dosing and distribution of any active is vital – it's just like medicine. Too little, and you'll not get the desired results. Too much, and you'll be at risk of side effects, without yielding any greater benefit.

Take care to avoid moving your active into areas you don't want it to go. For example, with your retinoid, avoid the eye area (for now) and lip area, and don't allow it to collect in any hollows, such as the sides of the nose or wrinkles. Otherwise, this will hurt in the morning.

HOW TO APPLY AN ACTIVE (THE DR SAM WAY)

In 2016, a patient who had consulted with me to tackle their pigmentation came back to clinic for follow-up. I had prescribed a topical regime and they were quite happy with their progress, but I spotted an issue – there was a visible line of demarcation along their hairline, where they had either missed a bit or applied their treatment unevenly. I realised there was a gap in how I'd instructed them to use their products, and devised my 13 Dot Technique as a result.

This simple principle serves two advantages: Firstly, you get an even layer all over without creating 'hot spots' where you deposit too much active and end up with sore, irritated skin. This gives a nice 'field effect' (when you improve the whole canvas rather than just focusing on a problematic chin, for instance). Secondly, it makes a tiny amount of active go a very long way, which is imperative when we're dosing ingredients, such as retinoids, which are very powerful. It's also economical.

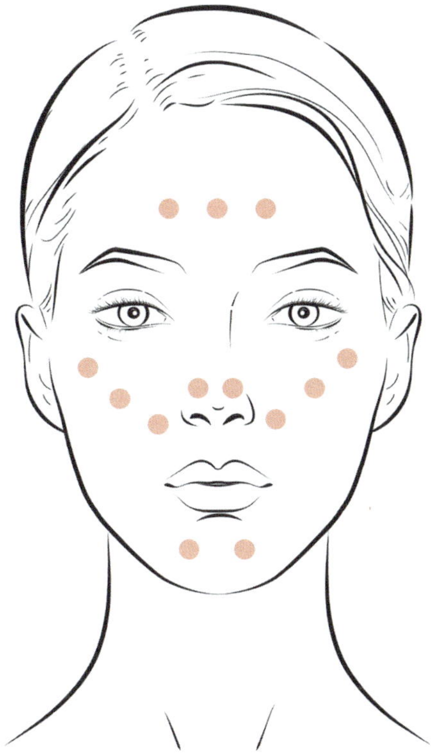

THE 13 DOT TECHNIQUE

1 Start with a pea-sized amount. Go and get a pea from the freezer to compare it to for the avoidance of doubt. More isn't better – it's just wasteful (and more likely to irritate).

2 Apply using the 13 Dot Technique:

- 3 dots across the forehead
- 3 on each cheek
- 1 on each side of the nose
- 1 on each side of the chin

This ensures even distribution and avoids overloading any one area.

3 Use your fingertips to connect the dots. Gently spread the product out and massage in fully. You want it to penetrate evenly. Blend well at the edges, like the hairline and jawline. Take care to avoid moving it into areas you don't want it to go (see box, opposite).

Zone your application if needed

If you are breakout-prone in the T-zone but dry around the cheeks, you can apply actives more selectively.

- Benzoyl peroxide or salicylic acid: apply just on the forehead, nose and chin. Don't just use on the individual blemishes; target the whole area which has *potential* to break out, so you get ahead of future problems.
- Retinoids or azelaic acid: apply over the whole face, but use less on reactive zones (for example the thin skin near the mouth).

Frequency matters more than quantity

Start with alternate-day use (or even every third day if your skin is very sensitive). On your days off, simply moisturize.

Establish a rhythm, then every two weeks, do a check-in with your skin barrier. See how your skin is behaving – if your barrier is happy, give things a nudge and increase the frequency to daily use. If that's okay after two weeks, try using a fingertip rather than pea-sized amount. Increase frequency first, then quantity.

Using the right amount regularly will always outperform overuse, which leads to barrier breakdown and the need for days off to recover.

BUFFERING

Buffering is a simple adaptation that really changed my practice when I first discovered it at a US conference. While for the most part we want to encourage product penetration, many of us have sensitive skin and this is more common as we age. An easy way to minimize the risk of skin irritation in the early days of your actives journey is to reverse the Activate and Hydrate steps in your routine. Moisturizing first slows down the penetration of your active and this helps protect your skin barrier while it becomes acclimatized. It also reduces the chance of error – by protecting thin skin around the mouth first, you vastly reduce the risk of waking up with a red, dry chin. Finally, when you are using a tiny amount of retinoid in the early days, it also helps give the skin a little slip, so it glides over the whole face more easily.

MOISTURIZER GOGGLES

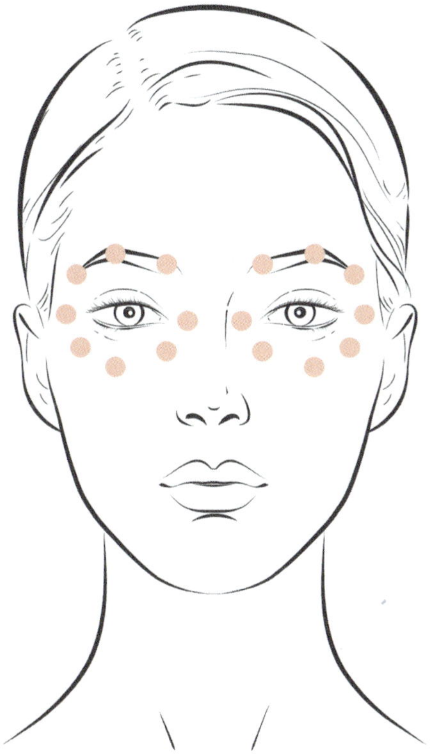

Moisturizer Goggles is a device I developed to help avoid what is perhaps the most common mistake someone is likely to make in the early stages of their actives journey. Gently apply moisturizer around the eyes to shield eye area from actives and prevent irritation.

NOTES FROM THE CLINIC

A patient started Epiduo (benzoyl peroxide and the retinoid adapalene in combination) at night and, like many do, applied it right before bed and went straight to sleep. Even though he avoided the eye area completely, the product hadn't fully dried down, and when his face smooshed into the pillow, it tracked towards his eyes overnight. He woke up with a puffy eyelid, red skin and a wave of panic, thinking he was allergic (he wasn't). This was a classic case of product migration. The fix? Moisturizer Goggles. Problem solved.

The moral of the story is that products can move around on your skin, however precisely they are applied. The solution is to intentionally 'block' the eye area with a generous layer of moisturizer before applying your active, to impede any transfer. It's also a good idea to wash your hands after applying your active before you go on to the next step: hydrate.

3 HYDRATE

If there's one step in your skincare routine that can dramatically impact the way your skin looks, it's hydration. The right moisturizer for you is one that contains the correct blend of ingredients to deliver long-lasting hydration and a skin finish and feel that's right for your personal taste.

The same moisturizer can be used in both your morning and nighttime routine, unless you prefer a different skin finish, in which case feel free to fine-tune accordingly. Some people like a lighter texture under their SPF during the day and a richer one at night for comfort.

A good moisturizer supports your skin barrier and at the same time helps reduce any irritation from your actives. It does not block their effectiveness when used correctly.

Hydration shouldn't feel like an afterthought. Get it right and you'll keep your skin looking plump, healthy and resilient every single day. Your make-up will last better and look fresher, too.

PILLING

Pilling occurs when skincare products roll off the surface of the skin in small, rubbery crumbs instead of being properly absorbed. A fingertip length is a good amount of product for the face.

Causes

- Applying too much product.
- Applying products to very dry skin, which increases friction.
- Not allowing adequate dry-down time between layers.
- Rubbing the skin too much during application.
- Layering incompatible formulas – often silicone-heavy products – on top of each other.

Solutions

- Use a smaller amount.
- Apply products to slightly damp skin, let them settle then pat or press products in rather than rubbing.
- Allow 30–60 seconds between layers.
- Make sure textures are compatible (lighter → richer).

HOW TO APPLY MOISTURIZER

1. Allow actives applied after cleansing to be fully absorbed. This ensures they stay where you've placed them, thus avoiding accidental movement to places they're not intended to go. This shouldn't take more than a minute and skin should feel touch-dry.

2. Move straight on to your hydration stage. You don't want your skin to dry out – you want to apply moisturizer while your face is still a little damp from cleansing to lock moisture in and avoid that dry, tight feeling.

3. Use the right amount. Too little and it won't provide adequate support; too much and it can interfere with layering and cause pilling (see box, opposite). Spread it over the areas of the face where you feel you need it, including the eye area if you're not using a designated eye cream. You may not need much on your nose if you have an oily T-zone (most of us do) and you may need more on your cheeks. On cold days you may need more; on humid days you may need less. Be responsive to what your skin needs.

4. Apply it with purpose. Gently smooth the moisturizer over your skin using fingertips with a sweeping motion to encourage absorption. Think of it as a gentle hug for your skin.

5. Don't forget your neck. Necks need love too. Use a similar fingertip amount and sweep it down to keep the skin here hydrated and smooth. And do not forget your décolletage. The science is unambiguous: what you do for your face should extend, without exception, to your décolletage. Thinner, drier and less sebaceous than facial skin, it accumulates photo ageing at an accelerated rate, so take the same diligent approach as you do with your face.

4 PROTECT

The most common error in skincare is probably underdosing SPF.[vii] There are many reasons for this: an unpleasant texture; a white cast that makes skin look odd; or a finish that disrupts make-up application. Or it may be due to vague guidance such as 'apply generously'.

The only way you get the full level of UVA and UVB protection is by applying a specific amount. Every sunscreen is manufactured using the standard testing amount of $2mg/cm^2$.[viii] The SPF on the label is only accurate at this thickness. It's a surprisingly large amount and it's common to underdose by as much as 25–50 per cent.

You might ask at what age sunscreen becomes a necessity. My advice is to start using sunscreen as soon as building a skincare routine is on your radar. Any teen using products to tackle blemishes will be using a retinoid. That means daily sunscreen is needed – it reduces the darkening of post-blemish marks further and, if skin is irritated from actives use, avoids aggravation from UV rays.

Protection for darker skins

Sunscreens for darker skins should ideally protect against visible light, not just UV (see page 85). The most useful ingredient for this purpose is iron oxide, the main ingredient used to tint colour cosmetics – by adding it to a sunscreen formulation, you end up with a handy hybrid that provides both protection and coverage.

SUNSCREEN REAPPLICATION

Good (office/mostly indoors)

- Apply the correct dose in the morning as your final skincare step. Allow it to set for one to two minutes.
- If applying make-up, use a Beautyblender to press cosmetics into the skin rather than rubbing, in order to avoid disturbing the film.

Better (on the go/active lifestyle)

- Morning application, plus a top-up every two hours when outdoors.
- Wear tinted sunscreen and keep colour cosmetics minimal so you're free to reapply through the day.

Best (beach/high-UV days)

- Reapply every two hours without fail and always after swimming, sweating or towel-drying.
- Use a water-resistant formula, wear a UPF hat and avoid UV between peak hours of 11am–3pm.

THE 3 DS

These are the keys to correct daily sunscreen use.

1 Dose

In practice, you need about 1.25ml (¼ teaspoon) of sunscreen for the average face. You need the same again for your neck. I urge you to go to the kitchen and see what a ¼ teaspoon dose looks like. It's more than you think, especially if you're using an SPF with a runny texture (I'm not a fan of SPFs in pipette format for this reason). I recommend you use a texture that makes it easier to visualize the correct dose, so you know you're doing it right.

2 Distribute

This is another place my 13 Dot Technique pays off. We don't want to miss areas like the eyelids, ears and around the hairline. That's why I don't believe in moisturizers with sunscreen in them. We want to apply moisturizer just where we need it – if we did this with our SPF, it would lead to disastrously inadequate and patchy sun protection.

3 Daily

This is the most powerful habit in skincare for preserving skin's youthfulness, if you start it early enough. Its benefits compound over time, just like interest. As with any habit, you want it to be automatic, just like brushing your teeth. If it's morning, the rule is sunscreen goes on in the correct dose with the correct distribution. This removes the mental effort of making a decision as to whether it's needed – remember, it's not just for sunny days.

THE EYE AREA: ITS OWN ZONE

The eye area is one of the first places to show signs of fatigue, early ageing and sensitivity.

The eye area demands careful consideration for several reasons. The skin here is up to five times thinner than the adjacent skin on the cheek; it's drier due to fewer oil glands and more susceptible to the impact of constant movement than anywhere else on the face. It also continues to thin with age, which is why it's one of the first places to show signs of fatigue, early ageing and sensitivity. Even brief, accidental contact with actives – such as a stray swipe of your retinoid – can be enough to trigger irritation. So, what does the eye area really need? It's simple: the same four steps as the rest of your face, and gentle handling.

During the day, our goal is to preserve skin thickness and elasticity. That means reaching for antioxidants and daily SPF to protect our collagen and elastin. So often the eye area is skipped when

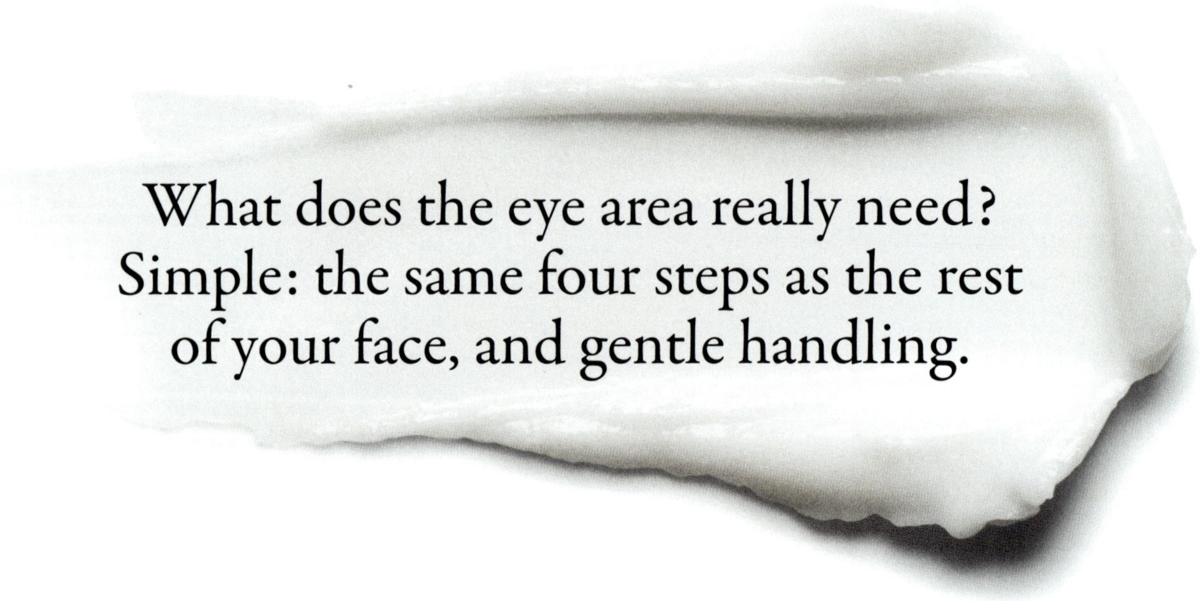

What does the eye area really need? Simple: the same four steps as the rest of your face, and gentle handling.

applying SPF and yet it's crucial if we're to protect our most vulnerable skin. My preference is to use a hydrating mineral sunscreen as it won't sting your eyes, permitting application close to the lash line.

At night, the focus shifts to building resilience. We can use the same actives we use elsewhere on the face to boost collagen, brighten tone and thicken skin over time; we simply need to manage their potency conservatively to minimize the risk of irritation.

Technically, you can use your regular moisturizer around your eyes – and for many that's adequate if the skin barrier is healthy and your concerns are minimal. But as you start to layer in actives and target specific issues (such as fine lines and dark circles), the eye area benefits from its own strategy. This helps deliver targeted actives at safe concentrations, while respecting the fragility of this zone.

Dark circles are something of an inevitability for most of us. Some of us are born with them, thanks to genetics and inherited pigmentation patterns. As we age and the already-thin skin around our eyes gets thinner still, darker structures such as blood vessels and muscle fibres underneath become more visible. Post-inflammatory hyperpigmentation (PIH) from rubbing, irritation or conditions such as eczema can also darken the area, particularly in darker skin tones. And lifestyle plays its part, too: poor sleep, dehydration and seasonal allergies all make circles more prominent.

A word of warning: some concerns in the eye area are beyond the realm of skincare. I'm talking about bags, droopy eyelids, hollowing and significant puffiness. These reflect structural changes beyond the skin that are best addressed by an experienced oculoplastic surgeon if they are a bother.

DO I NEED AN EYE CREAM?

If you adopt the Four Pillar approach (see page 76), I think that a routine that's correctly structured with the eye area's needs in mind can absolutely work. But it comes back to the principles of using the right ingredients, in the right combination, at the right concentration. It is less about using an eye cream per se and more about sourcing actives at the right level of potency for them to be beneficial without doing harm.

Most problems in the eye area that are most effectively managed by skincare are directed at boosting collagen, preserving skin thickness and maintaining elasticity. Avoiding inflammation is also critical, as even minor friction or irritation can trigger post-inflammatory hyperpigmentation (PIH). Use of actives must be tempered by barrier support and careful dosing.

Hydration makes a big difference to how fine lines in the eye area appear, by smoothing surface texture and improving how the light bounces off the skin, although it won't alter existing fine lines beyond this temporary effect. But that's okay – we have our retinoid for that.

Practically, you might want to use an eye cream that combines your Activate and Hydrate step in one to minimize layering in the morning – a good thing if we want our concealer to apply smoothly.

NOTES FROM THE CLINIC

Patients are often very concerned about their eye area, but are equally worried about using a retinoid on this delicate skin. I've found the greatest success comes from staggering the introduction of a retinoid around the eyes until after tolerance has been achieved on the rest of the face first. This way, confidence will have been gleaned (no doubt, after a few early errors) so that this advanced step can be easily mastered. I'd also recommend introducing one active at a time – so try vitamin C first in your morning routine, then a retinoid after a few weeks if that goes smoothly. I will also always drop the strength of retinoid – so even if someone is using a prescription retinoid on the rest of their face, I'll use a non-prescription retinoid on their eye area and always buffer with moisturizer first (see page 126). Granactive Retinoid 2% is a favourite as it's well tolerated. Likewise, retinaldehyde 0.05% is a good place to begin. The rules of increasing strength here are the same as for the rest of the face (see page 98).

AN EFFECTIVE ROUTINE FOR THE EYES

STEP	PRODUCT	AM	PM	APPLICATION	NOTES
Cleanse	Gentle cleanser Eye make-up remover (if needed for mascara and eyeliner)	✓	✓ ✓	Fingertips only Dampen cotton pad – press and wait 10 seconds before swiping. Don't rub.	Tubing mascara is a good idea if you have watery eyes, as it won't run and it slides off easily with warm water and gentle pressure.
Activate	Vitamin C Niacinamide	✓ ✓		Apply a thin layer along the bony orbit. Press into skin, don't rub. Do not apply to the more mobile skin of the eyelids.	Use 5–10% strength or stick to a gentle derivative (see page 115). This can easily be formulated within your moisturizer or SPF for fewer steps.
Activate	Retinoid		✓	Apply a thin layer along the bony orbit. Smooth and press into skin with your fourth finger for precision, don't rub. You need no more than a grain of rice amount for *both* eyes. Start using every third day and increase to alternate days after two weeks. Then use daily after two weeks.	Buffer with moisturizer first initially to protect the delicate skin and also create a little slip, so you can use a tiny amount of retinoid. Do not apply to the more mobile skin of the eyelids. There should be no excess to rub in – if there is, you've used too much.
Hydrate	Moisturizer	✓	✓		
Protect	Mineral SPF	✓			

MORNING VS NIGHTTIME ROUTINE

The purpose of our morning skincare routine is quite different to that of bedtime.

Let's look at our morning routine first. During the day, our skin faces a constant barrage of environmental challenges such as UV radiation, pollution and stress. These factors generate reactive oxygen species (ROS), the internal rust we explored in Chapter 2 (see page 40), which drives inflammation and the cumulative damage behind premature ageing, pigmentation and loss of firmness.

A nighttime routine looks quite different. Away from the threat of UV, our skin shifts into repair mode. Barrier function is restored, damaged DNA is repaired and cell turnover accelerates. This is the circadian rhythm at work.

AM

Your use of morning actives will be dictated by what you are trying to achieve. If it's a routine geared towards blemishes, your priority is controlling those, so ingredients such as salicylic acid and azelaic acid will be top of the list. If you're concerned about fine lines and pigmentation, it will be vitamin C and niacinamide.

These very different demands of day and night form the basis of how we structure a skincare routine, and much of that structure is anchored in the use of actives.

PM

Your PM routine is simple: a retinoid ALWAYS goes on the skin at night. This makes life easy, because it means that other actives generally get deployed as part of your AM routine. This one active is the most powerful part of your routine, make no mistake. We use retinoids at night partly because this is when your skin shifts into repair mode, but also because most retinoids are unstable in UV light. Unless they are intentionally co-formulated with other ingredients (like Epiduo), you don't need much else in your routine – just cleanse and hydrate. Choose a moisturizer that will help support your skin barrier with ingredients such as ceramides, which will help make tolerating your retinoid easier. There are a few exceptions to this – if you have an inflammatory skin condition, such as active rosacea or eczema, or if you're pregnant. But otherwise, a retinoid should be your PM priority.

ADAPTING THIS FRAMEWORK TO YOUR SKIN

A lot of anxiety exists around finding the right routine for your skin, but my actives-focused approach makes life very simple.

Let's take the example of a patient who has acne and some post-acne marks but a tendency to sensitivity. They've tried lots of acne products but found them all too harsh. Invariably, this kind of patient is product-hopping and winding their skin up by doing too much.

I focus on streamlining the 'support system': a simple cleanser, a niacinamide-enriched moisturizer and a sunscreen that won't clog pores. I might suggest a lighter-textured moisturizer for the morning and a richer one for nighttime. It's the job of these products to make using actives both easy and successful. I'll pair these with a gentle retinoid to clear pores and prevent breakouts; then I'll add in azelaic acid for its anti-inflammatory properties and to help tackle any dark marks.

On the following pages, I'll show you how I would formulate a routine in the clinic depending on your skin concern: what I'd consider, what I'd leave out, and how to build and adapt your routine for the best results.

HAVE I GOT SENSITIVE SKIN?

Most people who think they have sensitive skin actually have 'sensitized' skin. The symptoms are similar: stinging, burning, blotchy redness, feeling tight and dry. However, sensitive skin is a trait you're born with. Sensitized skin is a state you've created, often through barrier damage, and it can usually be reversed.

Your skin is probably sensitized if:

- The reactivity is recent, not lifelong.
- You can trace it to a new product, a more aggressive routine or a stressful life period.
- Your skin stings on application of products it used to tolerate.
- Your skin always feels tight or dry.

Your skin may be sensitive if:

- It has always reacted easily, even as a child.
- You have a personal or family history of eczema, rosacea, asthma or hay fever.
- Your skin reacts to temperature changes, wind or spicy food, not just skincare.

Not sure? Strip back to a simple barrier repair routine with no actives for 4–6 weeks. If the reactivity resolves, you have your answer.

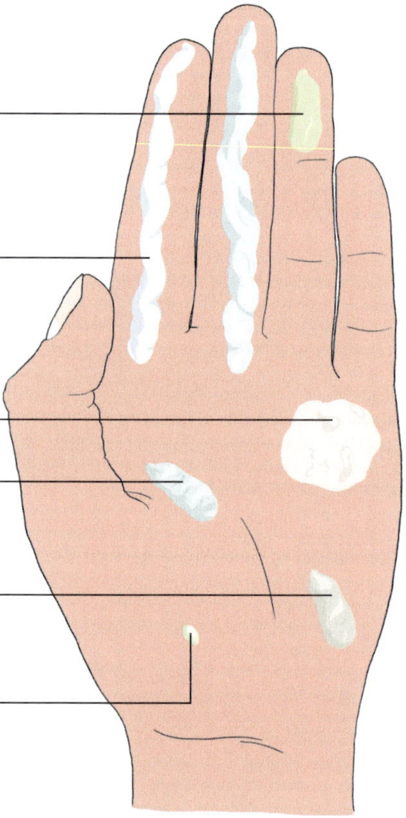

PRODUCT AMOUNTS

1 ACNE, CLOSED COMEDONES AND PIH

PHASE 1: ACTIVE INFLAMMATION

STEP	PRODUCT	AM	PM
Cleanse	Gentle cleanser	✓	✓
Activate	Salicylic Acid or Benzoyl Peroxide	✓	
Activate	Retinoid		✓
Hydrate	Moisturizer	✓	✓
Protect	SPF	✓	

PHASE 2: PREVENTION

STEP	PRODUCT	AM	PM
Cleanse	Gentle cleanser	✓	✓
Activate	Azelaic Acid	✓	
Activate	Retinoid		✓
Hydrate	Moisturizer	✓	✓
Protect	SPF	✓	

In the early stages, when inflamed blemishes are the focus, salicylic acid or benzoyl peroxide (BPO) in the morning help calm them, while your retinoid gets to work at night. As the inflammatory component settles, the focus shifts to preventing new comedones from forming and tackling Post-Inflammatory Hyperpigmentation (PIH). This is where azelaic acid takes over in the morning, with your retinoid continuing at night. Keep a spot treatment (benzoyl peroxide or salicylic acid) on hand for any new blemishes that break through.

2 REDNESS

PHASE 1: CALM AND STABILIZE

STEP	PRODUCT	AM	PM
Cleanse	Gentle cleanser	✓	✓
Activate	Azelaic acid	✓	build to ✓
Hydrate	Moisturizer (barrier-supportive)	✓	✓
Protect	SPF (mineral)	✓	

PHASE 2: INTRODUCE RETINOID

STEP	PRODUCT	AM	PM
Cleanse	Gentle cleanser	✓	✓
Activate	Azelaic acid	✓	
Hydrate	Moisturizer (barrier-supportive)	✓	✓
Activate	Retinoid (low-strength, buffered)		✓
Protect	SPF (mineral)	✓	

PHASE 3: FULL ROUTINE

STEP	PRODUCT	AM	PM
Cleanse	Gentle cleanser	✓	✓
Activate	Vitamin C	✓	
Activate	Azalaic acid	✓	✓
Hydrate	Moisturizer (barrier-supportive)	✓	✓
Activate	Retinoid (low-strength, buffered)		✓
Protect	SPF (mineral)	✓	

Redness-prone skin needs patience. Start with azelaic acid once a day, building to twice daily as your skin tolerates it. This is your foundation: anti-inflammatory, effective against background redness, and well tolerated by most.

After 3 months, if your skin is stable, consider introducing a retinoid at night (stopping azelaic acid use at night). Start low, go slow, and always buffer – the retinoid comes after your moisturizer in this routine, not before.

After a further 3 months, if things are going well, you can add vitamin C in the morning before your azelaic acid. This is the full routine, but there's no rush to get there, and you can stop and sit tight at any point. Each phase should feel comfortable before you move on.

3 PREMATURE AGEING

STEP	PRODUCT	AM	PM
Cleanse	Gentle cleanser	✓	✓
Activate	Vitamin C	✓	
Activate	Retinoid		✓
Hydrate	Moisturizer	✓	✓
Protect	SPF	✓	

This is the simplest routine of all these, and for many people it's where they'll start. Vitamin C in the morning protects against oxidative damage and supports collagen. Your retinoid at night does the heavy lifting on repair and renewal.

Niacinamide doesn't need its own step here. Look for it as an ingredient in your moisturizer or SPF, where it works quietly in the background, reinforcing ceramide production and supporting your barrier without adding another layer to your routine.

4 PIGMENTATION

STEP	PRODUCT	AM	PM
Cleanse	Gentle cleanser	✓	✓
Activate	Vitamin C	✓	
Activate	Azelaic acid	✓	
Activate	Niacinamide	✓	
Activate	Retinoid		✓
Hydrate	Moisturizer	✓	✓
Protect	SPF	✓	

Pigmentation responds best to a multi-checkpoint approach. Vitamin C, azelaic acid and niacinamide work together in the morning to interrupt melanin production, transfer and calm inflammation. Your retinoid at night accelerates cell turnover, helping to clear excess pigment that's already there. SPF is non-negotiable here; no combination of actives will outwork inconsistent sun protection when your melanocytes are the problem.

5 PREGNANCY

STEP	PRODUCT	AM	PM
Cleanse	Gentle cleanser	✓	✓
Activate	Azelaic acid	✓	✓
Hydrate	Moisturizer	✓	✓
Protect	SPF	✓	

No retinoid, please. Discuss anything else you're using on prescription with your doctor before continuing. For those with acne, this can seem an alarming prospect. However, I find that if your acne is well controlled prior to stopping – and I recommend stopping your retinoid as you start actively trying to conceive – alternative safe and effective ingredients can be combined so that control is maintained.

Azelaic acid carries the routine here, working in both the morning and evening to manage common concerns such as breakouts, redness and the pigmentation that pregnancy hormones love to stir up. Niacinamide can be built into your moisturizer or SPF for extra barrier support. If breakouts flare, salicylic acid at concentrations up to 2% and benzoyl peroxide as a spot treatment are both safe options. And feel free to add in vitamin C for extra glow and assistance on the pigmentation front. Your retinoid will be waiting for you on the other side.

When you have a concise toolkit of actives that really work, tweaking a routine for different scenarios and skin concerns is straightforward.

USING ACTIVES FOR MENOPAUSE

Menopause is defined as the point one year after a woman's last period. On average, it occurs at the age of fifty-one. There are a host of physical changes that accompany its onset, many of which start gradually in your forties (the perimenopause). When it comes to our skin, two major things happen: firstly, the skin thins and we lose a lot of collagen – as much as one-third of our stores disappear in the first five years, so anticipating this is crucial.

Secondly, oestrogen helps skin retain moisture, so when levels plummet, skin becomes dry and reactive. The skin's microbiome also becomes less diverse, compounding the problem. This is a conundrum: we need actives to maintain our skin's scaffolding, but it won't tolerate them as easily as before. We therefore need to plan our routine carefully with these changes in mind.

While the collagen-building benefits of a retinoid or vitamin C are clear, we need to mitigate the risk of irritation with moderation of their strength, frequency and formulation, choosing lower concentrations, gentler derivatives and barrier-supporting bases. Niacinamide is immensely helpful here. It offers an ideal balance, supporting collagen production in its own right while reinforcing ceramide production to help offset the skin changes driven by oestrogen depletion. Buffering is also indispensable (see page 126).

A WORD ON TEEN SKIN

Rising hormones means more oil, bigger pores and breakouts. The instinct is often to attack these symptoms with harsh cleansers and scrubs. This tends to backfire; stripping the barrier triggers irritation, which can worsen breakouts and, in darker skin tones, cause more marked post-inflammatory hyperpigmentation (PIH).

A teen routine with mild acne needs just 4 products: a gentle cleanser, one active for breakouts (salicylic acid or benzoyl peroxide), a lightweight, non-clogging moisturizer, and SPF every morning. That's it. Keep it simple, keep it consistent.

To be clear: teen skin does not need anti-ageing skincare. Vitamin C serums and elaborate multi-step routines are unnecessary and can do more harm than good on young, healthy skin. An over-the-counter retinoid is the logical next step if there are persistent clogged pores or breakouts, but this is for managing congestion, not for anti-ageing.

If breakouts are scarring, painful or not improving after 2–3 months, see a dermatologist. Early treatment prevents damage that is far harder to reverse later.

SUMMARY

As you can see, when you have a concise toolkit of actives that really work, tweaking a routine for different scenarios and skin concerns is straightforward. It's simply a case of flexing the routine around your actives to support their use.

If you keep cleansing simple, that flex largely comes from your Hydrate step. I often encourage patients to have two moisturizers on the go at a given time: one for drier days and one for oilier days.

Skin is dynamic, after all. Some nights you'll not sleep well and skin will be drier. In summer, the higher temperature and humidity means it might well be oilier. The framework stays the same. It's only the details that shift.

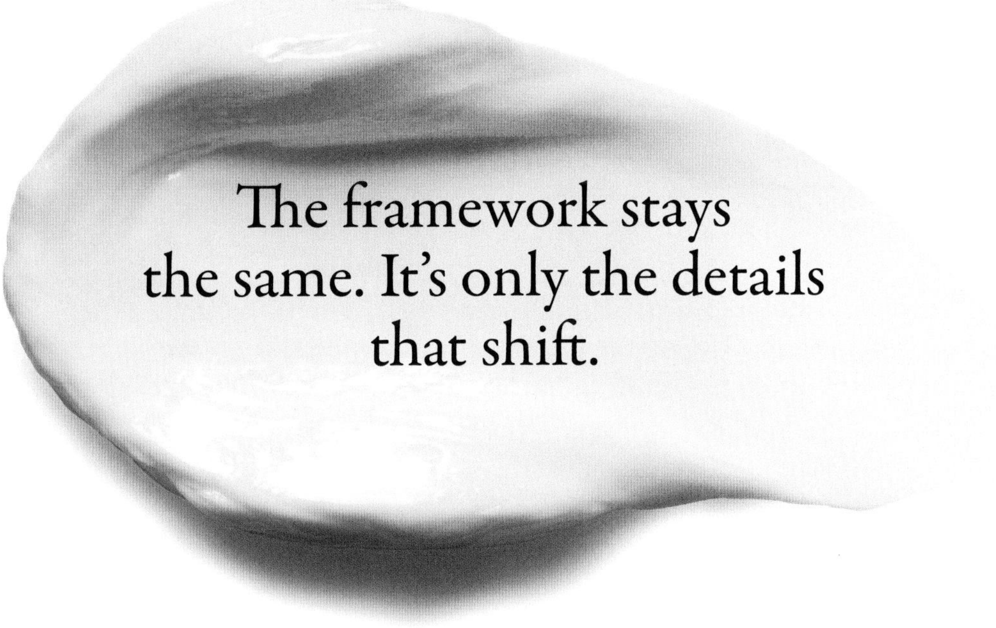

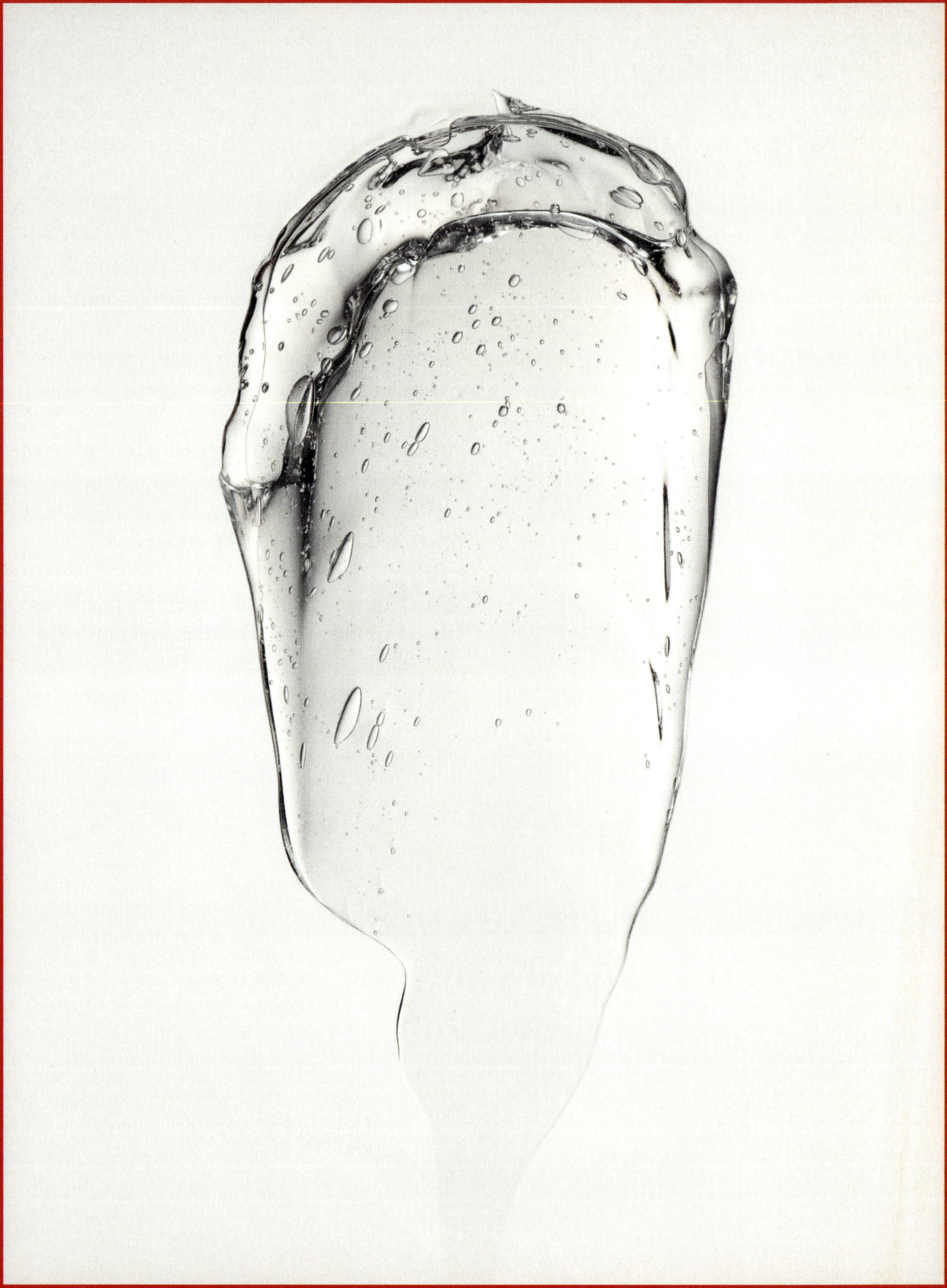

7

Finding the Right Products for YOU

HOW TO DECODE PRODUCT LABELS AND MARKETING CLAIMS

By this point you should be able to label your key skin concerns, have decided whether your skin is sensitive or not; have nailed your actives; and have got your Four Pillars in order!

The big question now is: what on earth do you buy? Standing in the busy aisles of the pharmacy, decision fatigue can hit hard.

Most of us don't want or need a shelf full of skincare. What we do want is the ability to cut through the noise, decode the label and select what will *actually* serve our skin. Think of this chapter as your real-world shopping guide to what really matters.

The INCI list is the part that cannot lie.

THE INCI LIST DEMYSTIFIED

Flip over a bottle of any serum and you'll be confronted by a list of ingredients that will make your toes curl. It's usually printed so small you'll need a magnifying glass (and possibly a chemistry degree) to decipher it. But fear not. This mysterious jumble of Latin and lab-speak is called the INCI list, short for International Nomenclature of Cosmetic Ingredients. It sounds intimidating, but in reality this list is your secret weapon. No matter what the front of the bottle says ('clean', 'natural', 'dermatologist-approved', 'clinically proven'), the INCI list is the part that cannot lie. It tells you what's inside . . . kind of.

The INCI list is skincare's version of a recipe. It's a standardized list that shows exactly what's in a product and in what relative amounts. Ingredients are listed in descending order by weight, until you hit the 1% line, meaning the ingredient present in the highest concentration comes first and the smallest amounts are found at the end. After that, brands can list ingredients in any order they like.

The first four to six ingredients typically make up about 80 per cent of the formula. So, if a brand is shouting about niacinamide or vitamin C on the front of the bottle, but those ingredients are buried near the end of the INCI list, allow your inner sceptic to arch a brow. It means there's barely a dusting of the active ingredient you're paying for. It's like buying a chocolate-chip cookie and discovering there's only one chip.

Armed with these facts, you can work out a lot, even if the product itself isn't transparently labelled with the percentages of key active ingredients.

The goal is to spot the green lights and the red flags. A common sleight of hand in skincare marketing might go like this: a shiny, exotic-sounding new ingredient is positioned front and centre – a rare alpine flower, perhaps, or a molecule harvested from volcanic ash. The name is novel, the story seductive. But if you turn the bottle around, you'll often find a familiar heavyweight, like retinol, anchoring the formula and doing much of the work. It's not that the new ingredient has no merit – it might, it might not – but the true results you see in the mirror are often owed to the tried-and-tested stalwarts. Knowing how to decode the INCI list lets you see past the sparkle and get to the substance.

RED FLAG

If the ingredient you're looking for appears after fragrance (often added at just 0.1–0.5%), it may be present in a very low concentration – possibly too low to deliver meaningful results. Some actives do work well at low doses, but if a hero ingredient is trailing behind parfum, it's worth questioning the claims.

BEHIND THE BUZZWORDS

Don't be fooled by marketing claims – let's look behind what some of those buzzwords really mean.

1 'DERMATOLOGIST TESTED'

This means what it says: a dermatologist was involved in testing the product, but the exact nature of the testing isn't defined or indeed regulated. There's no industry standard. For example, it may involve a dermatologist supervising patch testing on a small group (number unclear) of people to check for irritancy (outcome unspecified). In other words: vague.

2 'CLINICALLY PROVEN'

Things improve a bit here. A clinical protocol of sorts was used and results produced would be statistically significant (and therefore were unlikely to occur by chance). But the term is again unregulated, so when you dig deep, you'll often find that a tiny number of people were in the study, it was conducted in-house and it might only report consumer perception (such as '85 per cent said their skin felt smoother after four weeks').

That's quite a different scenario to the way we approach credible evidence in medicine, where studies are blind-tested, powered to achieve statistical significance, done independently and peer-reviewed to remove bias, with clear endpoints, such as a percentage improvement in acne lesions.

3 'NON-COMEDOGENIC'

This is a term that tells you that a product was formulated in a way that shouldn't clog your pores. There is no standard or required testing for a product to be certified non-comedogenic. Nowadays, we no longer use animal testing, so what this means is your INCI list is scrutinized by a safety assessor working with your formulator to exclude ingredients known to clog pores, such as isopropyl myristate or coconut oil.

My personal stance on this is that a product labelled non-comedogenic has at least been formulated through the lens of doing no harm when it comes to acne-triggering potential. This is a good place to start. If you know your skin is easily clogged, do a patch test (see page 151) on a small area of clear skin first.

4 'CLEAN BEAUTY'

This is a popular but unregulated marketing term that typically refers to products free from certain ingredients that are perceived as harmful, such as parabens or synthetic fragrances. While it suggests safety and purity, the reality is that every brand or retailer defines 'clean' differently, often using fear-based messaging that vilifies ingredients with strong safety records. Natural doesn't always mean better. Nettles are natural – that doesn't mean they're good for your face.

'Clean' doesn't guarantee a product is effective, non-irritating or well formulated. In fact, several well-known brands have had their 'clean' products pulled from the shelves due to preservative failures and microbial contamination. This can pose a serious health risk, particularly for those with a compromised skin barrier concern, such as eczema. It's the very opposite of clean.

KEY CATEGORIES YOU'LL SPOT ON EVERY INCI LIST

Here's what you'll find on most labels, and what each category does:

- **Base ingredients** (usually water/aqua): come first.
- **Humectants** (eg glycerin, hyaluronic acid): pull water into the skin.
- **Emollients** (eg squalane, fatty alcohols): soften and smooth.
- **Occlusives** (eg petrolatum, dimethicone): lock hydration in.
- **Actives** (niacinamide, retinoids, salicylic acid, azelaic acid): biologically active compounds that change something in the skin.
- **Preservatives** (phenoxyethanol, sodium benzoate): keep the product shelf-stable, stopping it from cultivating a microbial invasion.
- **Fragrance and essential oils**: improve the sensorial experience, but can be potential irritants, especially in sensitive skin.
- **pH adjusters** (eg citric acid, sodium hydroxide): maintain skin-compatible pH and formula stability.
- **Solvents** (eg propylene glycol, alcohol): help dissolve other ingredients or improve penetration.

HOW TO COMPARE PRODUCTS USING THE INCI LIST

This is a useful exercise if you're searching for a specific ingredient but are overwhelmed by choice. Let's take an example: you want to compare two niacinamide serums. Here, it's important to know your benchmarks. For niacinamide, the ideal strength is somewhere between 5–10%. Above 10% won't necessarily improve efficacy, but might lessen tolerability. Below 2% and it's doubtful much will happen.

Look at where niacinamide falls on the list. Is it in the top three (likely at a strength of at least 5–10%)? Is it midway down the list (likely 2–5% and therefore probably still effective)? Or is it at the bottom (less than 1%, so doing very little)?

Of course, there's more to a formula than any one ingredient. So you also need to look at whether it is supported by complementary ingredients that enhance its actions – for example, azelaic acid partners brilliantly with niacinamide to calm inflammation and improve skin tone. Are there any potential irritants (such as fragrance or unnecessary alcohol)?

Ultimately, this all becomes easier when you shop with brands that believe in transparency in labelling, as opposed to enigmatic-sounding proprietary complexes, where you have no idea what ingredient is doing what. This is more important than ever in today's landscape of

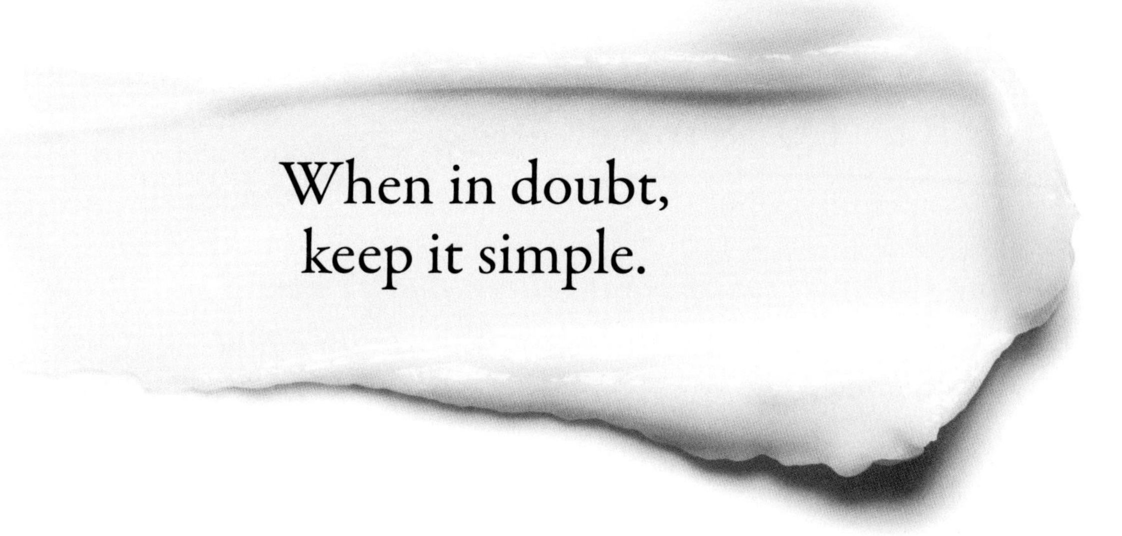

empowered, ingredient-savvy consumers. It helps build trust, improves results and enables you to avoid expensive mistakes.

APPROACH THE SKINCARE AISLE WITH CONFIDENCE

If you're new to decoding INCI lists, stick to products with shorter ingredient lists. Learn to recognize the key actives for your concerns and know their dosing sweet spot. Choose brands that are transparent and focused on performance.

Understanding the INCI list puts the power in your hands. It's how you move from confused to informed, and from product-hopping to building a skincare wardrobe that actually works.

Once you understand how to interpret an ingredient list, you gain the ability to assess a product based on its true merits, not just its claims. With this knowledge, you'll approach the skincare aisle with clarity and confidence, selecting formulations that align with your skin's needs.

PATCH TESTING 101

If you have sensitive skin, patch testing is a smart move. Apply a small amount of the product behind your ear or on your jawline, once daily for 3–5 days. Watch for signs of redness, stinging or irritation. If your skin stays calm, you're likely good to go. It's a simple way to avoid a full-face tantrum and builds confidence in a new addition to your routine.

WHEN TO SPEND, WHERE TO SAVE

Building a skincare routine that delivers doesn't have to mean blowing your budget. In fact, being savvy about what not to buy can free up resources to invest where it really counts. Here's how to make your money work harder, without compromising on results.

1 SKIP REDUNDANT CATEGORIES

Think you need a separate cream for your neck? Think again. High-quality facial products are perfectly suitable. Most 'specialist' creams offer very little beyond clever marketing, and investing here often leads to disappointment. Save your time, your money and your morale.

2 AVOID INGREDIENT DUPLICATION

It's surprisingly easy to double up on actives without meaning to. Many people unknowingly layer multiple retinoids in a single routine because they're focused on the marketing claims, not the ingredient list. A quick check of your INCI list will help you avoid unintentional overlap. Less is more.

3 CHOOSE MULTITASKERS

Efficiency is everything. The best products deliver multiple benefits in one elegant step. When active ingredients are blended synergistically at just the right levels, you get better performance than trying to cobble together a multi-layered routine on your own.

This principle applies beautifully to skincare/make-up hybrids, too. A well-formulated tinted sunscreen means you can skip foundation. A nourishing tinted lip balm eliminates the need for both lip colour and hydration. These simple swaps save time, energy and – yes – money.

4 DON'T SPLURGE ON CLEANSERS

I've expressed my preference for rinse-off, active-free cleansers, which means they don't spend much time on your skin. They should be functional and gentle, designed to do no harm. That's it. And you only need one. Double cleansing is unnecessary if your cleanser is doing its job properly.

5 INVEST IN A SUNSCREEN YOU LOVE

We know what properties to look for in our sunscreen. But at the end of the day, the only thing that will make you apply your sunscreen correctly at that $2mg/cm^2$ dose is loving its texture and finding it layers well with the rest of your morning routine. So, if it takes spending a bit more to find The One, that's a good investment.

6 THE DELIVERY SYSTEM MATTERS

Two serums can contain the same active at the same concentration and perform very differently. The reason is often the delivery system – the technology used to package and transport an active ingredient into the skin. Ingredients such as retinol and vitamin C are inherently unstable or irritating in their raw form. Modern formulations use encapsulation, liposomal technology or time-release mechanisms to protect the active and disperse it gradually into the skin. This improves both efficacy and tolerability. On a label, look for terms such as 'encapsulated', 'liposomal', or stabilized derivatives such as retinaldehyde or ascorbyl glucoside. A sophisticated delivery system may add to the price tag, but if it means your skin can tolerate an active it otherwise couldn't, that's money well spent.

3-MINUTE FORMULA CHECK

Here's how to size up a product fast:

1 Look for an anchoring active, based on your key concerns. The right ingredients, at the right concentration, in the right combination.

2 Identify any red flags. Is it over-promising? Does it contain possible pore-cloggers? Are there ingredients that are likely to irritate sensitive skin?

3 Determine if you like how it feels on your skin. Some of us like dewy, others love matte. It's personal.

SKIN FEEL

After the active ingredients themselves, skin feel is one of the most important features of your routine.

This might sound counterintuitive, but I believe it is an important consideration. In the early days of my clinical practice, I curated a carefully chosen selection of products so that every patient could leave their first appointment with a complete routine. Everything was fragrance-free, so I focused on products that delivered on the formulation first, of course, but texture was a close second. This became the mechanism for coding pleasure into my clinic protocols.

Skin feel is pivotal when building your morning routine, in particular our Hydrate and Protect pillars. These are the daily workhorses that matter because they determine skin finish and, if you're wearing make-up, they will contribute to how well it wears. If you have a product that pills or goes patchy, it's game over. It simply won't become a habit. The finish on your skin at night matters much less, because you're off to bed.

Trialling products in-store or buying travel-sized samples are good ways to assess this all-important aspect of any product. If you won't enjoy using it, it won't work – no matter how solid the INCI list.

DR SAM'S FAVOURITE INGREDIENTS FOR SKIN FEEL

TEXTURE	HOW IT FEELS	LOOK FOR ON THE INGREDIENT LIST
Cushiony	Plumping and luxurious	Cetearyl alcohol, stearic acid, cetyl alcohol
Velvety	Smooth, soft-focus, good slip	Dicaprylyl carbonate, caprylic/capric triglycerides, cetyl ethylhexanoate
Silky	Glides on to skin, no greasiness	Dimethicone, squalane, isohexadecane
Jelly-like	Juicy and bouncy	Carbomer, xanthan gum
Melts-in	Quick-absorbing, deeply comforting	Cetearyl olivate, sorbitan olivate, shea butter

POWER COUPLES

We've learned about the INCI list – what to look out for and what buzzwords are hype.

But there are some ingredients which work best in partnership with others. When you learn how to combine them, they can offer you powerful results that you wouldn't necessarily see from each ingredient on its own.

ACTIVE 1	ACTIVE 2	WHY THEY WORK TOGETHER	BEST FOR
Retinoid	Azelaic acid	Tackles pigmentation, smooths fine lines and delivers breakout control	Acne + PIH, melasma, ageing skin
Retinoid	Niacinamide	Niacinamide strengthens the barrier, helps reduce irritation and redness, boosts retinoid tolerance	Ageing skin, rosacea-prone, beginners to retinoids
Vitamin C	Niacinamide	Brightening + barrier support + antioxidant defence. Ideal for daily defence and glow	Dull, uneven skin tone, urban stressors
Benzoyl peroxide	Adapalene (Retinoid)	BPO tackles bacteria, adapalene prevents pore clogging	Moderate to severe acne, inflammatory breakouts
Azelaic acid	Vitamin C	Double-down on pigmentation, antioxidant and anti-inflammatory support	Rosacea with sun damage
Lactic acid	Niacinamide	Gentle exfoliation + hydration + barrier support	Texture, dehydration, sensitized skin
Salicylic acid	Niacinamide	Pore clearing meets redness reduction. Ideal for sensitive, acne-prone skin	Blackheads, large pores in blemish-prone skin
Bakuchiol	Vitamin C (THD or MAP)	Antioxidant protection + radiance boost without irritation	Sensitive skin, pregnancy-safe anti-ageing

8

Life Below the Neck

THE NEGLECTED AREAS OF SKIN

We tend to forget that the body deserves bright, clear skin too.

When we look at someone's face, we are unconsciously processing the quality of the neck, chest and hands at the same time. It's why many celebrity photos from the eighties, when tanning was at its peak, are so jarring – faces maintained with the utmost of care contrast with a décolletage that hasn't quite stayed in sync.

With so much focus on our faces these days, body concerns are rarely the main reason someone seeks an appointment with me. Having said that, at least one in five patients raise a body issue during the consultation at some point. It's always something I explore if someone is getting married, as body concerns require a plan and adequate time to tackle them, just as we would the face. When your gown is backless, discovering four weeks before the big day that a fresh breakout has occurred with all the last-minute stress is not relaxing.

Too often, we leave the body to fend for itself against decades of UV exposure, the odd sunbed session and reactive skincare habits. But with very little extra effort, we can create continuity from our faces to our feet by applying The Four Pillars, adapted for the body.

UNDERSTANDING THE TERRAIN: HOW BODY SKIN DIFFERS

Epidermal turnover (the natural process by which skin cells are produced, mature and shed) is significantly slower on the body than on the face. While facial skin typically renews itself every 28 days, areas such as the legs or arms may take up to 40–60 days. This slows down further as we age.

This means that older, less luminous dead skin cells accumulate more easily, leading to limbs that look dusty with dullness and skin that's scaly to the touch. It also means that actives, such as exfoliating acids or retinoids, may struggle to penetrate and results may take longer to become visible. Patience and consistency are required.

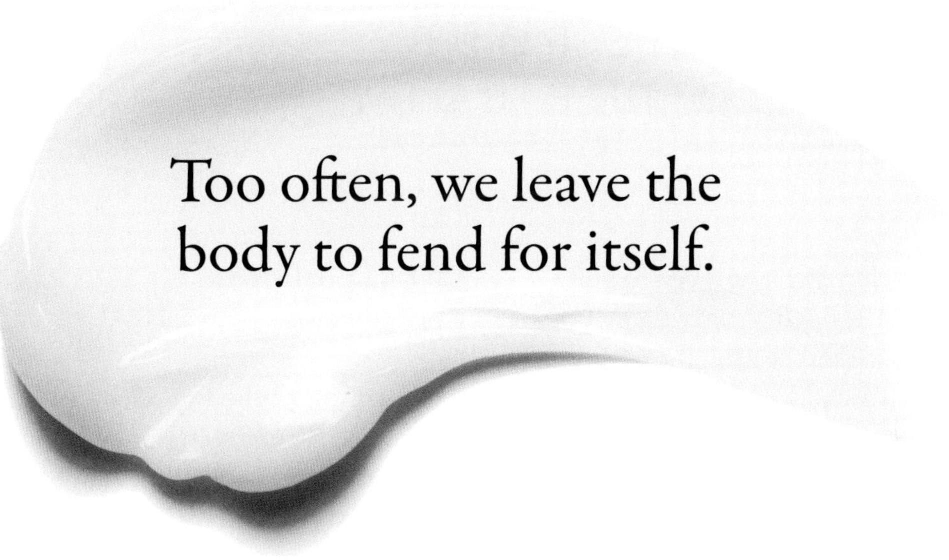

Too often, we leave the body to fend for itself.

This is compounded by a thicker stratum corneum in places like the knees and elbows. This provides more protection against friction and knocking into things (a good idea), but it presents a further challenge for product penetration.

Practically, this means we may need to formulate body products differently, using either higher concentrations of actives, or ingredients and strategies that enhance product penetration.

At the same time, the skin on the body has fewer sebaceous glands (chest and back aside), so you'll find that the limbs in particular are more prone to dryness and irritation if neglected, due to lower levels of sebum supporting the skin barrier.

Finally, our body skin is often incidentally exposed to the environment, meaning cumulative UV damage is inevitable unless thought about proactively. Think about how many times a day we wash our hands, depleting our skin barrier a little on each occasion; yet they're exposed to the impact of UV and pollution just as much as our faces are. If we neglect their care generally, and UV protection in particular, they will age at a very different rate.

APPLYING THE FOUR PILLARS TO THE BODY

We've talked before about how best to build habits that stick. It's vital to make them simple and achievable so that the habit forms through repetition. That's why I'm not going to ask you to do a four-step body routine twice a day. Think of this as a flexible framework you can scale up or down, depending on time, lifestyle and concerns.

1 CLEANSING: EVERYDAY ESSENTIAL

Cleansing the body is often rushed, squeezed between shampooing and shaving. Done with intention, it supports the skin barrier and microbiome. Choose a non-foaming, pH-balanced cleanser, just as you would for the face. If skin is dry or sensitive, skip anything with fragrance and stick to a short, tepid shower once a day, with a quick rinse after exercise if needed.

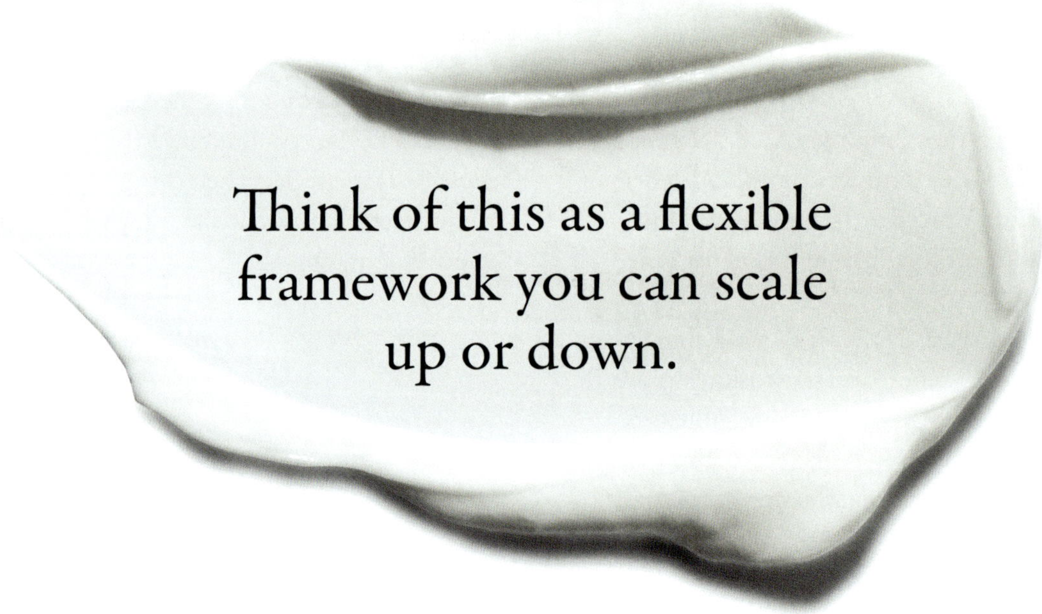

2 ACTIVATE:
DO YOU NEED ACTIVES ON YOUR BODY?

When it comes to using actives on the body, the key question isn't 'should you?', but 'where and why?'. Unlike the face, where actives often form the backbone of every routine, the body benefits most when ingredients are used with a targeted approach, where needed.

THE 2-MINUTE MOISTURIZING RULE

Moisturize within two minutes of getting out of the shower, while skin is still damp, to lock moisture into your skin barrier.

3 HYDRATE:
MOISTURE AS BARRIER SUPPORT

Most people only moisturize when they see dryness, but hydration is fundamental for healthy, resilient skin. The key is consistency with barrier-supporting humectants, emollients and occlusives in fast-absorbing formulas. Go fragrance-free if you're prone to irritation or pigmentation, and avoid pore-clogging oils on breakout-prone zones.

4 PROTECT:
YOUR BODY NEEDS PROTECTION, TOO

Don't forget to apply sunscreen to all exposed areas of skin – see pages 83–7 and 130–1 for more on SPF protection.

THE BIG 5 BODY ISSUES

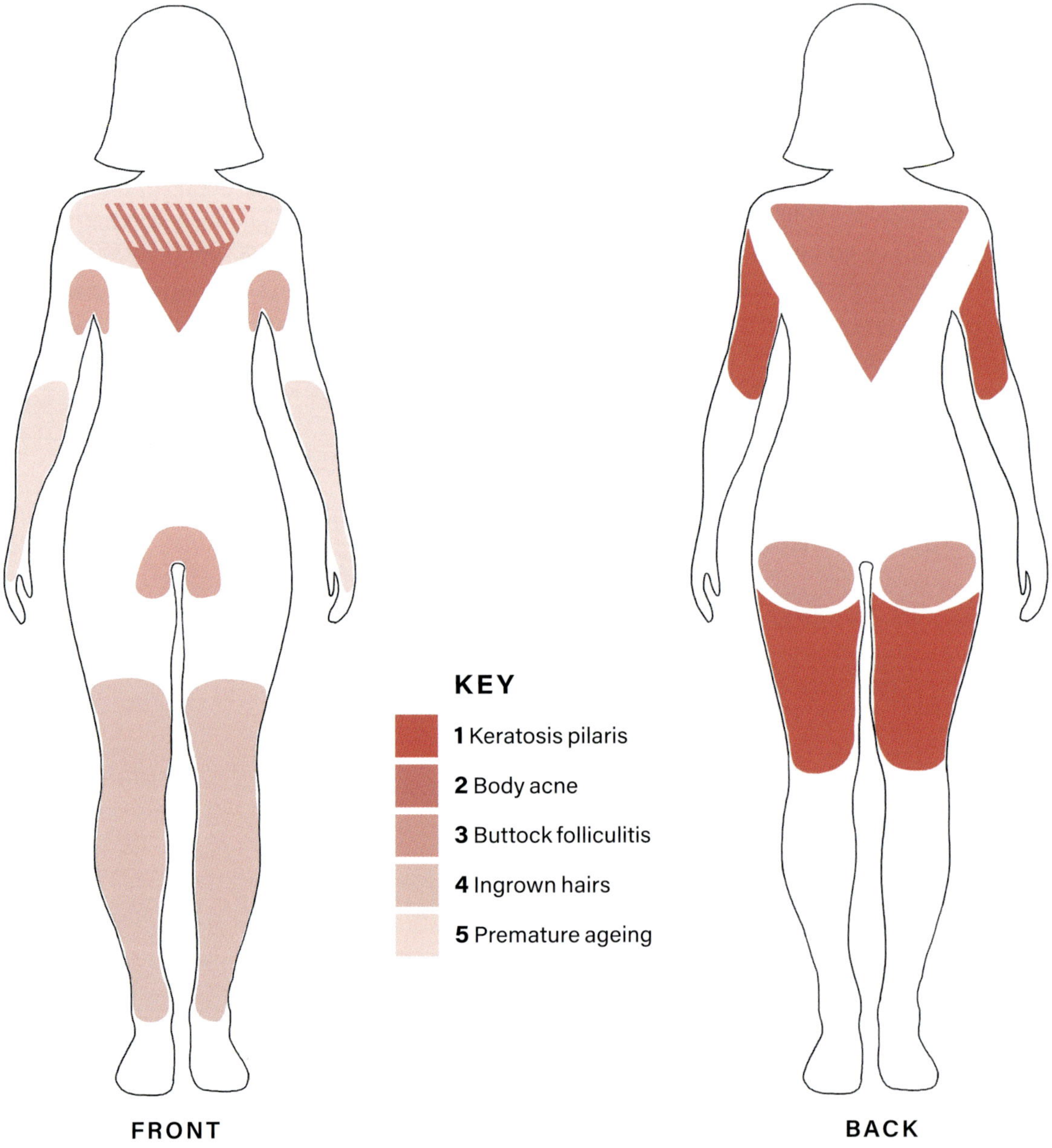

1 KERATOSIS PILARIS

This is probably the most common body issue I see (and one I have myself). It's so common that one in two of us carry the genes for it. In some individuals, there's nothing to see; in others, it shows up as a bumpy rash on the backs of arms and thighs. When you look closely, there's a little ball of keratin (which is the roughness you can feel) in the hair follicles, surrounded by a rim of redness.

2 BODY ACNE (OR 'BACNE')

Acne is the most common inflammatory disorder in the Western world and it can occur wherever there are lots of sebaceous glands. Around 50 per cent of those with facial acne will have involvement of the chest or back. Chests are sensitive and backs are hard to reach, so that can make treatment a bit of a challenge. Factor this into your plan.

3 BUTTOCK FOLLICULITIS (OR 'BUTT ACNE')

This is actually not true acne, as there's no comedone kicking off the problem. Instead, we see folliculitis on the buttocks where the hair follicles become inflamed. It's terribly common and something people are often quite embarrassed about. Sweat, heat and friction from clothing are at the heart of the problem – think sitting down in tight jeans all day. It upsets the microbiome within the hair follicles, facilitating overgrowth of less-friendly bacteria. This results in follicular inflammation and their signature pustules, so you see spots with white-topped red bumps that look a bit like acne.

4 INGROWN HAIRS AND HAIR REMOVAL PROBLEMS

Most forms of hair removal have some impact on the hair follicle too. Take waxing or epilation, for example. The physical impact of pulling the hairs out can upset the residents within the follicle, disturbing the microbiome, leading to red bumps. Shaving can cause cut hairs to retract into the follicle (especially if they're curly), where they coil up and get stuck, behaving like a foreign body. The immune system jumps into action to evict the intruder and a red, tender bump of inflammation develops to try to eliminate the hair. Other factors can make hairs more prone to becoming trapped in the first place – afro-textured hair, tight clothing, prolonged sitting and a lack of regular exfoliation all contribute to blocked exit routes for emerging hairs. Ingrown hairs are more than a cosmetic irritation; they can become chronically inflamed, leading to post-inflammatory hyperpigmentation or even secondary infection if they are picked or irritated repeatedly.

Even if hairs don't get stuck, the act of shaving itself is a form of intense exfoliation and the friction can trigger redness and discomfort, especially if the blade is dull and there's a lack of lubrication. Don't stretch the skin, and try using a single-blade razor to avoid cutting hairs too short (which allows them to more easily retract into the follicle and get stuck).

5 PREMATURE AGEING

Sun damage tends to insidiously accumulate on the décolleté, forearms and the backs of the hands – those sun-exposed areas that rarely receive the same level of protection as the face. Loss of collagen, damage to elastin and irregular clumps of melanin can all contribute to a crepey, discoloured appearance.

WHAT CAN WE DO ABOUT ALL THIS?

The good news is that body skin is usually very tolerant of actives, so we can be efficient (punchy even) when needed. Conveniently, most of the actives we use on the face can work just as hard for us on the body. We don't need a brand-new toolkit. Skin is skin.

Most of the actives we use on the face can work just as hard for us on the body.

Exfoliating acids, such as lactic, mandelic and salicylic acid, are brilliant for unclogging, smoothing and brightening in one fell swoop. Azelaic acid works wonders for pigmentation, bacne and follicular inflammation. For more advanced concerns, a retinoid can improve tone, texture and dermis density, especially on sun-worn skin.

TARGETED ACTIVES FOR SKIN CONCERN

CONCERN	ACTIVES	HOW THEY WORK
Keratosis pilaris	Lactic acid, glycolic acid, niacinamide	Exfoliate bumps, smooth texture, hydrate dry patches
Body acne	Benzoyl peroxide, salicylic acid, azelaic acid	Kill bacteria, clear pores, calm inflammation
Buttock folliculitis	Salicylic acid, benzoyl peroxide	Zap bacteria, reduce redness
Ingrown hairs	Lactic acid, mandelic acid, retinoids	Free trapped hairs by speeding up cell turnover, fade marks, keep follicular exits clear
Premature ageing	Retinoids, niacinamide, vitamin C	Boost collagen, firm skin, even tone

THINGS NOT WORTH LOSING SLEEP OVER

I'm a big believer in throwing energy at things that we can influence and forgetting about those we cannot. A kind of skincare stoicism, if you will.

- **Cellulite**
  Around 90 per cent of women have cellulite. It's a normal structural feature of the female form, rather than a flaw or a disease. By contrast, only around 10 per cent of men are affected by cellulite. Lots of treatments exist that promise smoothness – generally a sign that no single treatment works brilliantly. My advice is to make peace with it.

- **Stretch marks**
  Over the years I've witnessed patients try to address these and have seen very little evidence that anything makes a tangible impact. Time takes much of the colour away, but if stretch marks are very bothersome, lasers can help expedite this. Nothing significantly impacts the indented silvery appearance, as this is an elastin problem, which we're not good at fixing. File them under 'leave them be'.

ACTIVATE: WHAT TARGETS WHAT

We can actually begin the work of activation on the body with our cleanse – it's simply efficient.

You may recall that I like to keep facial cleansers active free. The body is more forgiving, as there's no delicate eye area to navigate and it generally has more tolerant skin; actives in a cleanser make good sense here. Exfoliating acids offer a quick win, whether we use beta hydroxy acids (BHAs) to tackle bacne, or alpha hydroxy acids (AHAs) to tackle keratosis pilaris, ingrown hairs and premature ageing.

Product formats to consider

- **Lotions:** For speedy absorption on the limbs.
- **Sprays:** For tricky-to-reach areas such as the back.
- **Gels:** For better spreadability (especially on hair-bearing areas).
- **Roll-ons:** For underarms.

How to apply

When applying actives as part of a cleanser, leave it on the skin for a minute before rinsing. This is a kind of 'mini-mask' technique we call 'short contact therapy' in dermatology. It helps to deliver even, more effective results.

THE BODY SKINCARE PYRAMID

This is a useful way of applying the principles of The Four Pillars (Cleanse, Activate, Hydrate and Protect) in a way that's practical for the body, from daily essentials at the bottom to targeted actives at the top.

How to use the pyramid

- Do the **base steps** (Foundation: Essentials) every day (Cleanse + Hydrate).
- Add the **middle step** (Protect) whenever you're exposed to UV light. This is the long-term investment step that pays dividends over decades, preventing sagging, pigmentation and crêpiness. Regularly exposed areas need daily protection, whereas the rest of the body can be protected as needed.
- Sprinkle in the **top step** (Targeted Actives) only where and when you need it. Often this can be built into cleansing or hydrating products, so it doesn't add extra steps.

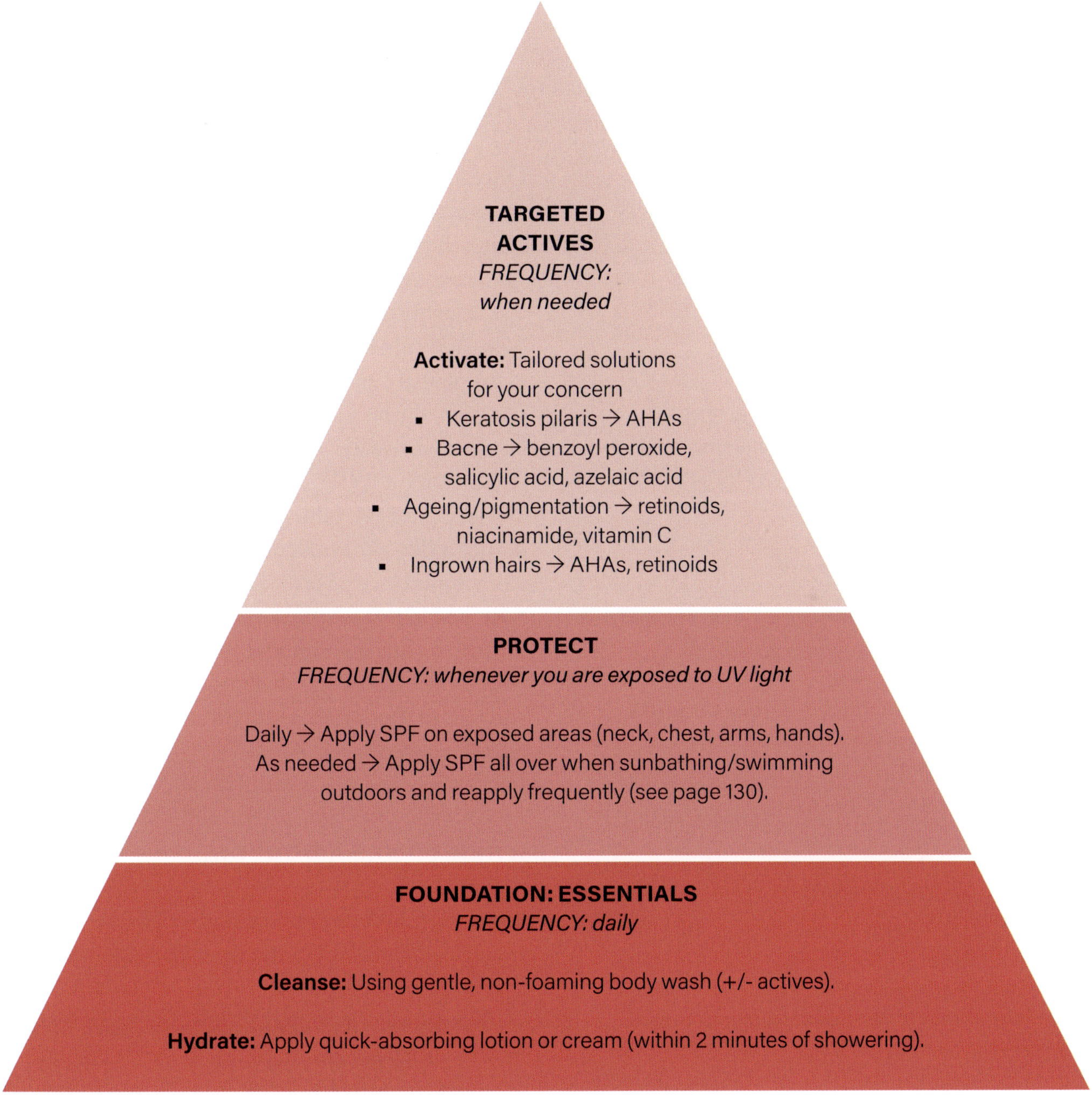

THE BODY SKINCARE PYRAMID

SPECIAL CONSIDERATIONS FOR DARKER SKIN TONES

Darker skin is naturally thicker and more compact, which means it can hold on to dull surface cells longer, but it also has a **heightened risk of post-inflammatory pigmentation (PIH)** when irritated. This is as true for the skin on the body as it is on the face.

The secret is **gentle consistency**. Hydrating exfoliants such as **lactic and mandelic acid** are ideal: they lift dull cells while pulling water into the skin, leaving it smooth and luminous.

Avoid harsh scrubs and overly strong peels; friction and inflammation are the enemy. The goal isn't to assault the epidermis; it's to keep it compact, hydrated and light-reflective.

Melanin-rich skin often has lower ceramide content, so hydration is vital after any exfoliation step.

THE FORGOTTEN ZONES: THE CHEST AND HANDS

Once we have the face under control in clinic, my attention often turns to what I call the forgotten zones: the neck (see page 129), chest and hands. These are among the areas most exposed to the elements throughout life and are therefore especially vulnerable to photoageing. Yet while many of us are meticulous about caring for our faces, the neck, chest and hands are often overlooked, usually in that order.

The goal is for everything to match. These areas should follow the same core principles as the face: daily sunscreen whenever exposed, with regular reapplication, proven active ingredients such as vitamin C, niacinamide and a gentle retinoid where tolerated, alongside appropriate cleansing and barrier support. If you're investing in your face, don't stop at the jawline.

WHEN TO SEE A DOCTOR

Most body-skin concerns respond well to the strategies in this chapter. But if you notice folliculitis that keeps returning despite treatment, spots that are becoming deeply inflamed or painful, signs of infection such as spreading redness, warmth or pus, or any changing moles or new growths, don't delay – see your GP or a dermatologist.

PROTECT: THE FORGOTTEN STEP

When it comes to the body, sunscreen is still treated as optional.

Most people wouldn't dream of skipping SPF on their face, but when it comes to the body, sunscreen is often reserved for beach days, holidays or heatwaves. But UV exposure is happening all the time, particularly if you live in a warm or sunny climate. From the moment you step outside – whether it's walking the dog, loading the car, or popping out on your lunch break – your skin is absorbing UV radiation. And let's not forget that UVA rays penetrate glass, so even that quick drive to work or the school run becomes another moment of cumulative exposure.

The key to making daily SPF a non-negotiable habit is making it friction-free. Choose a formula that dries down quickly, doesn't stain or stick to clothes, and layers effortlessly with the rest of your routine. Consider keeping a sunscreen in your gym bag, at your desk, or by the front door. Anything that removes 'I forgot' from the equation. Also, don't underestimate the power of visual prompts. Placing body sunscreen next to your facial one makes it far more likely you'll use it.

AT THE BEACH

When outdoors for a significant amount of time, we need to expand our Protect pillar to ensure all exposed skin is properly cared for. As I said in Chapter 4, getting the dose right is *by far* the most important factor in using SPF correctly.

SUNSCREEN DOSE PER BODY SITE

1 teaspoon for each arm

2 teaspoons for each leg

1 teaspoon for the chest

1 teaspoon for the back

I urge you to teach yourself what this dose looks like using an *actual* teaspoon with your sunscreen of choice. Practically, I find creams are a lot easier to dose and apply accurately. Watery lotions can be tricky simply because they run everywhere, and sprays, while appealing, deliver an unpredictable amount to the skin. Experience tells me that if a mechanism of sunscreen application seems too good to be true (watery, pipette-dispensed, moussey), then you're probably in danger of under-applying.

Combine sunscreen with a hat and body-covering clothing (both should have a high UPF rating), and seek shade during the hours of 11am–3pm to minimize exposure when UV rays are at their peak.

ONCE-DAILY SUNSCREENS

Single-application sunscreens are a thorny topic. A number of sunscreens bill themselves as adequate for a full day's sun without reapplication. Fantastic idea. Alas, this is not something I can recommend. If you're by the beach, you'll be sweating, swimming and likely towelling your skin. All of these actions can wipe sunscreen away, leaving skin vulnerable. So, please treat this type of sunscreen like your usual one and reapply regularly.

Your skin is the largest organ in your body.

A WORD ON SELF-TANNING

Self-tanning creams use something called dihydroxyacetone (DHA) to produce a temporary staining of the skin. I am a big fan of the self-tan. Firstly, it's the only safe version of tanning. Secondly, it's one of the best ways to camouflage things we can't really change on the body, like the ruddy hue on the backs of the arms in keratosis pilaris.

However . . . there is a challenging aspect to self-tan, aside from simply learning how to put the stuff on without streaking. If you are acne-prone, it may trigger closed comedones and breakouts. Whether this is due to DHA itself or other ingredients, such as odour-masking oils, in the self-tan is not clear, but I've seen it often enough to mention it here.

I advise patients to do their fake tan application in the early evening, where possible, so they can wash it off before bed. Kinder to the sheets, kinder to the pores. This also allows a corrective treatment regime to be applied overnight. Ingredients that speed up cell turnover will mean that the tan might not last as long, but if you regularly reapply a gradual tanner and build up colour slowly over a few days, you should find this is a manageable way to have your cake and eat it.

Your skin is the largest organ in your body, yet we often treat the face and body as though they are separate entities. In an ideal world, the appearance of your skin would be seamless from head to toe, so I hope I've convinced you that the time spent caring for the skin below your neck is just as important as the time spent caring for your face. Small daily choices, even just two minutes in the shower spent intentionally, can make a big difference in your journey towards bright, clear skin from head to toe.

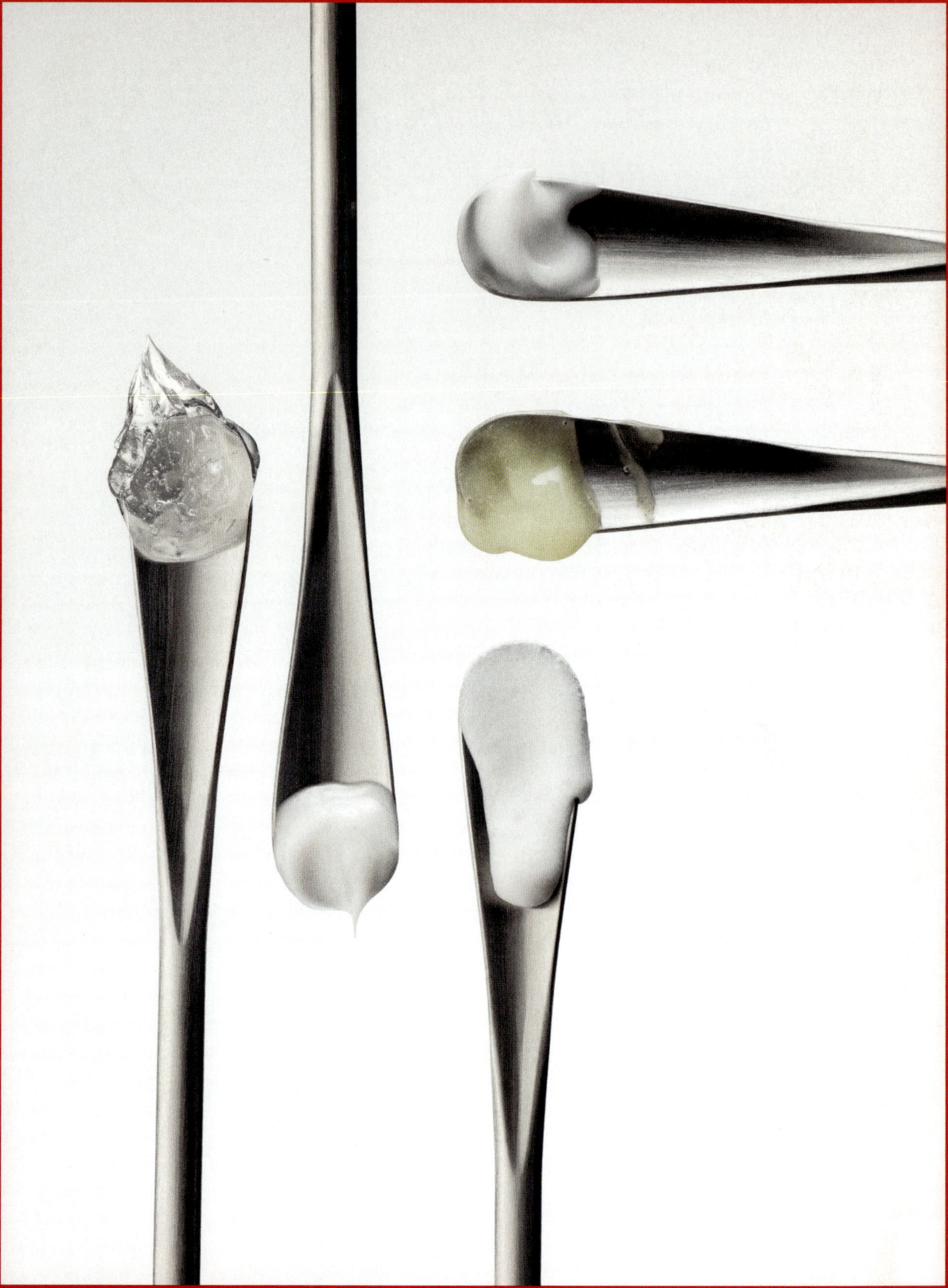

9

The Future of Skincare

PREJUVENATION

Congratulations! You've come a long way in understanding how your skin truly works.

You've learned how skin protects itself, how it responds to stress and inflammation, and how damage accumulates over time. But what if skincare didn't have to wait for visible problems to appear? What if we could support skin function early, intervening at a biological level rather than simply carrying out surface correction?

This shift towards prevention, resilience and longevity is shaping the future of dermatology. Known as prejuvenation, it reflects a growing focus on preserving skin health rather than repairing decline.

We've already explored how external stressors accelerate ageing from the outside in. Now, we turn inward. This isn't anti-ageing – undoing damage that's already been done. This is age-proofing – maintaining skin health and preventing further decline.

What if we could support skin function early, intervening at a biological level rather than simply carrying out surface correction?

THE CELLULAR STRUCTURE OF BRIGHT, CLEAR SKIN

Our understanding of how skin behaves has deepened dramatically in recent years.

We now know that many visible skin concerns begin long before they reach the surface – rooted in cellular processes that determine how well skin defends itself, repairs damage and renews over time. Understanding these mechanisms allows us to intervene earlier, more intelligently and with far-reaching consequences for long-term skin health.[ix]

MITOCHONDRIAL HEALTH

We've already covered the central role that reactive oxygen species (ROS) and oxidative stress play in driving skin ageing (see pages 29 and 40) – the internal rust sparked by UV exposure and pollution. What's important to understand is that oxidative stress doesn't only come from the outside world; it's also generated naturally within the skin itself.

Inside every skin cell is a vast transport network responsible for delivering energy exactly where it's needed. Rather than thinking of mitochondria as static 'power stations', imagine them as trains running along a network of tracks. Each train represents the cell's ability to generate usable energy, while the tracks represent the cellular infrastructure that allows that energy to be delivered efficiently. When this system is working well, skin cells have the energy they need to defend themselves, repair daily damage and regenerate. That vitality shows on the surface as clarity, resilience and glow.

But energy production comes at a cost. As these trains run, they naturally generate sparks – reactive oxygen species. In small amounts, these sparks act as useful signals inside the cell, themselves triggering necessary renewal and repair. In fact, this is how the system is designed to work.

The challenge is that the majority of oxidative stress in skin is generated internally by mitochondria themselves, so there isn't much reserve in the system. When too many sparks build up, they begin to damage the tracks. Damaged tracks lead to faulty trains, which generate even more oxidative stress, and things go downhill from there. When UV exposure and pollution add further oxidative stress to a system at breaking point, the network begins to falter. Energy delivery becomes unreliable. Repair slows. Collagen production drops. Over time, this breakdown becomes visible as loss of firmness, dullness, barrier dysfunction and premature ageing.

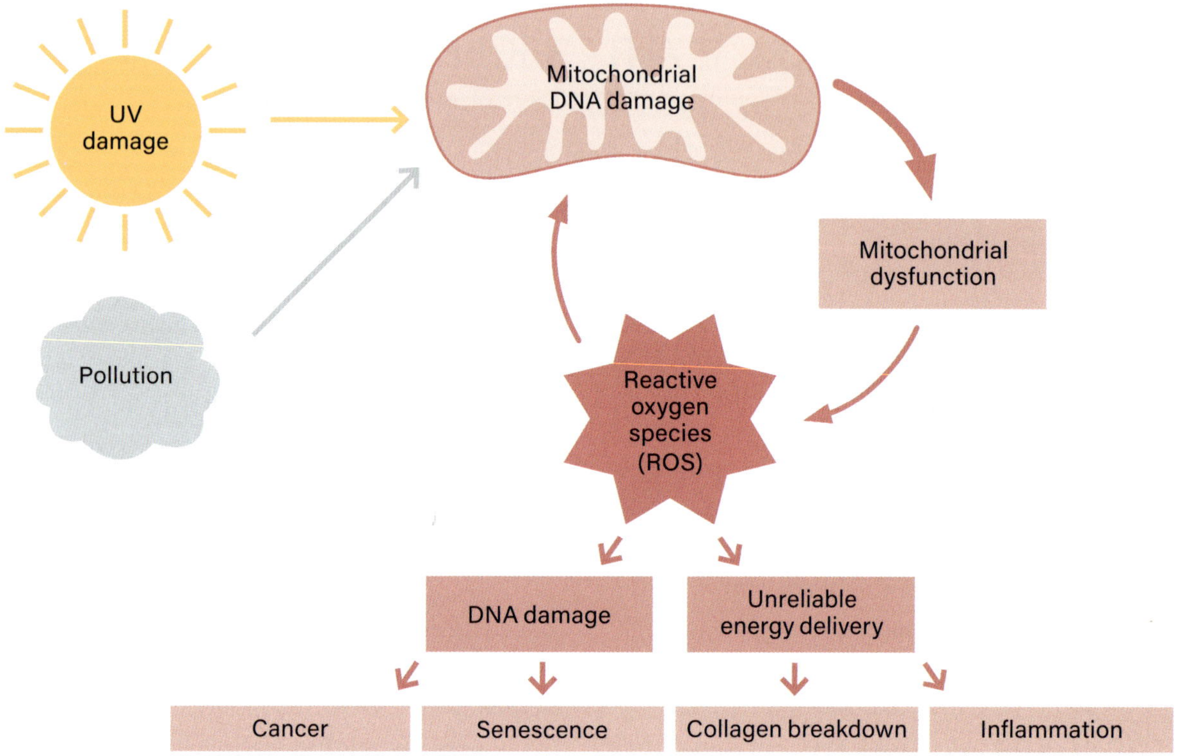

THE VICIOUS CYCLE OF OXIDATIVE STRESS

NAD+ DEPLETION

For this transport system to run smoothly, the trains need fuel. That fuel is NAD+ (nicotinamide adenine dinucleotide), a vital coenzyme required not only for generating energy, but also for activating the repair pathways that fix DNA damage and maintain cellular housekeeping. This is the link between cellular energy and cellular repair. When NAD+ is plentiful, both systems work. When it's depleted, both suffer.

As mitochondrial efficiency declines, more NAD+ is consumed simply to keep the system running. Less is left over for repair. By around the age of 40, NAD+ levels have fallen to roughly half of what they were in childhood.[x] When oxidative stress occurs, those already-depleted reserves drop even further. The result is a cell that struggles to recover.

In real terms, this means skin tires more easily. Redness lingers longer. Healing slows. Radiance fades faster. The trains are still running, but the fuel gauge is permanently low.

WHAT IS NAD+?

NAD+ is a coenzyme that's present in every living cell in every living thing – from bacteria to blue whales to you. Without it, cellular energy production stops within seconds. It is as fundamental to life as oxygen, yet many people have never heard of it. NAD+ drives the reactions that turn food into fuel, repairs DNA damage as it accumulates, and coordinates the proteins that govern how well and how fast we age.

CELLULAR SENESCENCE

When energy shortages and DNA damage persist, some cells reach a critical threshold and enter a state known as cellular senescence. Our cells aren't designed to live forever. Under normal circumstances, damaged or ageing cells are programmed to shut down and be removed through a controlled process called apoptosis.

Sometimes, however, instead of quietly bowing out, damaged cells take a middle path. They stop dividing, keep their structure and remain metabolically active. These are senescent cells, sometimes called 'zombie cells' because they're neither fully alive nor truly dead and they can spread their dysfunctional state to their neighbour.

In youth, this is a clever safeguard. Keeping these cells in place maintains tissue structure until the immune system clears them away. But with age, clearance slows. Senescent cells accumulate, and their inflammatory output, known as the senescence-associated secretory phenotype (SASP), begins to disrupt healthy neighbouring cells.

Energy failure, impaired repair and NAD+ depletion are all triggers for this process. Senescent cells then worsen the picture further: they are heavy consumers of NAD+, drawing down the reserves that healthy neighbouring cells depend on.

SENESCENCE AND AGEING

Senescent cells, or 'zombie cells', are damaged cells that have stopped functioning properly but don't die when they should. Instead, they remain in the skin, releasing inflammatory substances that harm neighbouring healthy cells. Over time, their accumulation can accelerate visible skin ageing.

THE BIG PICTURE

When mitochondrial trains slow, fuel runs low and senescent cells accumulate – the consequences ripple outward. Collagen and elastin degrade. The skin barrier weakens, allowing irritants and microbes to penetrate. Pigment regulation falters, driving uneven tone and stubborn pigmentation. Inflammation becomes chronic. What begins as a cellular energy problem becomes the familiar signs of visible ageing.

As we untangle the biology of ageing, it's increasingly clear how mitochondrial dysfunction, NAD+ decline and cellular senescence are deeply connected. The most forward-thinking skincare of the future will address them together, making bright, clear skin a possibility at any age.

MEASURING WHAT MATTERS

If the damage that drives ageing is invisible and accumulating years before a single wrinkle appears, how would you ever know where you stand? This is where the work of Professor Mark Birch-Machin gets genuinely exciting. His team has spent nearly three decades studying mitochondrial DNA damage in human skin and has developed a simple, non-invasive skin swab that can quantify it. Because mitochondrial DNA is so vulnerable to UVA and lacks the repair systems that protect your nuclear DNA, it accumulates damage in a way that is both measurable and meaningful.

Think of it like a blood pressure reading for your skin. You can't feel high blood pressure, but it's silently damaging your heart. Once you detect it through screening, you can do something about it and track whether what you're doing is working. This test does the same thing for your skin – it captures a snapshot of your skin's stress over the previous month, a barcode of cumulative damage.

This technology is already being used by aesthetic clinics to validate skincare claims with real biological data. But the bigger prize is putting it into the hands of consumers. Imagine tracking the impact of your sunscreen or retinoid over six months, not by scrutinizing before-and-after photos but by measuring what's happening at a cellular level. That is prejuvenation in action: intervening early, measuring objectively and adjusting course based on evidence.

EMERGING ACTIVES

Now that we understand the interplay between mitochondrial dysfunction, NAD+ decline and cellular senescence, we need new tools to help bring these processes back under control.

While The Four Pillars remain the foundation of healthy skin, skincare science doesn't stand still. A new generation of ingredients is emerging that aims to support skin at its biological roots, enhancing energy production, protecting mitochondria and managing cellular clutter. A note of honesty: these actives are promising but they don't yet have the breadth of long-term clinical evidence that we see behind a retinoid or vitamin C. We're still in the early chapters of this story. What follows is where the field is headed.

RECHARGING THE CELL: BOOSTING NAD+

Given the fundamental role of NAD+, it might seem logical to apply it directly to the skin in order to restore its youthful levels. Unfortunately, NAD+ is a large, unstable molecule that cannot easily penetrate the skin barrier and breaks down readily when exposed to heat and light. Instead, skin cells are equipped with specialized pathways that allow them to manufacture and recycle NAD+ internally, as long as they're supplied with the right building blocks. These can be provided internally from the blood stream by the diet or they can be supplied by skincare from smaller, more stable precursor molecules (such as niacinamide) that can penetrate the skin and be converted into active NAD+ exactly where it's needed, if conditions are right.

Sunflower shoot extract (SSE) is an intriguing discovery in this area. The young shoot, which must defend itself against environmental stress before the plant is fully developed, is densely packed with energizing metabolites. In skin, SSE supports mitochondrial function and activates the same NAD+ recycling pathway as exercise, one of the most powerful mechanisms we know for addressing age-related decline.

Oral NAD+ precursor supplements such as nicotinamide mononucleotide (NMN) and nicotinamide riboside (NR) have generated great interest, but their role is beyond the scope of this book. Topical delivery has the advantage of targeting skin cells directly, at the site where they're needed.

PROTECTING THE POWERHOUSES: MITOCHONDRIAL GUARDIANS

Just as any transport system requires maintenance, mitochondria need protection to function efficiently. A growing number of ingredients are being studied for their ability to safeguard these organelles and optimize energy flow.

- **Coenzyme Q10** supports the mitochondrial electron transport chain, improving energy efficiency and reducing oxidative 'leak'. This makes the trains run faster and cause less collateral damage in the process.
- **Pyrroloquinoline quinone (PQQ)** and **mitoquinol (MitoQ)** stimulate mitochondrial biogenesis, encouraging the production of new, healthier mitochondria. That translates to more tracks for trains to run on.
- **L-carnitine** and **alpha-lipoic acid** support fatty acid transport and redox balance within the cell. This again helps the trains to run fast.

Together, these ingredients help keep energy delivery reliable, inflammatory noise low, and skin function resilient.

Mitochondria need protection to function efficiently.

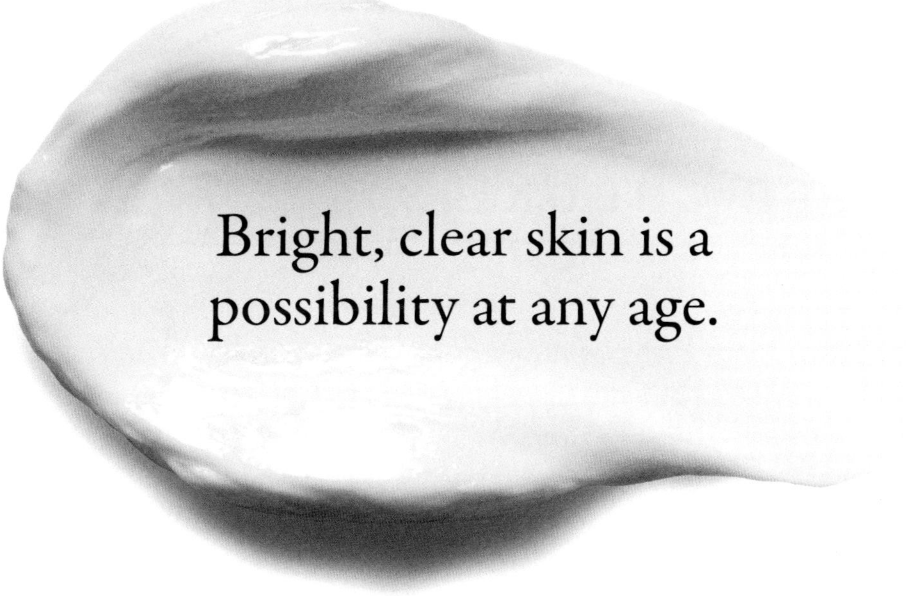

CLEARING THE CLUTTER:
TARGETING SENESCENCE

Fibroblasts are the collagen-producing workhorses of the dermis. When healthy, they maintain the structural scaffolding that keeps skin firm and elastic. When exposed to repeated oxidative stress or energy shortages, they can enter senescence.

Emerging senotherapeutic ingredients aim to address this cellular clutter, either by encouraging the removal of senescent cells (senolytics) or by suppressing their inflammatory output (senomorphics).

- **Silybum marianum** (milk thistle extract) acts as both a senolytic and a senomorphic, helping clear worn-out fibroblasts while calming inflammatory signalling.
- **Fisetin**, a flavonoid found in fruits such as strawberries, helps reduce the senescent cell burden and restore collagen integrity.
- **Apigenin**, derived from chamomile and parsley, gently reprogrammes senescent cells to behave better, protecting surrounding tissue from further damage.

Crucially, by addressing problems upstream, we stay true to the FLAWLESS principle of simplicity. It's about using fewer products, chosen more intelligently and sequenced more effectively, allowing your existing Four Pillar routine (see page 76) to work even harder.

When skin has the energy and capacity to respond, retinoids can activate their instructions to our genetic programmes more effectively, antioxidants can neutralize oxidative stress more efficiently, and barrier repair becomes faster and more resilient. In understanding these invisible forces, we stop chasing lines in the mirror and start caring for the machinery of youth itself.

THE MITOCHONDRIA-FRIENDLY LIFESTYLE CHECKLIST

Mitochondria don't work in isolation. They are social organelles that help us sense and adapt to the world around us.

They communicate, form networks and respond collectively to signals from the environment. Everything on the list below is a conversation with that network. Sunscreen reduces the oxidative burden on mitochondria that are already working hard to keep skin cells repaired. Exercise stimulates mitochondrial renewal across tissues, including in the fibroblasts that build our collagen. Sleep gives the network time to restore itself. Small, consistent habits build up over time because our mitochondria are constantly listening.

Daily defence

- Apply sunscreen every morning to limit the oxidative burden on your skin.
- Use antioxidant skincare (Vitamin A/C/E, bakuchiol) to give support to your skin's inbuilt antioxidant defences.
- Calm inflammation (azelaic acid, niacinamide) to reduce the signalling that depletes NAD+.
- Boost NAD+ and protect mitochondria (SSE + niacinamide), supporting energy production at its source.
- Use a retinoid and supplement with senolytics to support cellular renewal.
- Cleanse at night to remove pollution residue that generates ongoing oxidative stress while you sleep.

Smart nutrition

- Eat a Mediterranean-style diet that is rich in fruit, vegetables, oily fish and olive oil. This provides a broad base of antioxidants and anti-inflammatory compounds.
- Include lycopene-rich foods such as tomatoes and watermelon, which go further to support internal antioxidant reserves.
- Enjoy polyphenol-rich drinks and food, such as green tea, coffee and dark chocolate, to support mitochondrial function.
- Top up your NAD+ levels with tryptophan-rich foods such as poultry and bananas, and niacin-rich foods such as salmon, tuna and mushrooms.

Movement and metabolism

- Exercise regularly (ideally a mix of cardio and strength) to boost new, healthy mitochondria, not only in the muscles but *also in the fibroblasts*, leading to more collagen and thicker skin. Exercise also activates NAD+ recycling.

What matters most is consistency and clarity.

- Consider intermittent fasting – being a little bit hungry can be good for us. Try fasting for up to 16 hours by eating within an 8-hour window. This encourages autophagy, a kind of cellular clean-up operation, to stop energy wastage and improve cellular efficiency.

Rest and recovery

- Get consistent, high-quality sleep. This allows DNA repair to happen away from the harmful influence of UV, prompts the release of melatonin (a powerful antioxidant) and allows NAD+ levels to replenish. It also aids energy conservation as our heart rate lowers and our temperature drops.
- Manage stress consistently. Chronic cortisol release depletes antioxidants and suppresses tissue repair. Regular practice of relaxation techniques, such as meditation or breathwork, supports mitochondrial resilience.
- Use short, well-managed bursts of controlled thermal stress (hormesis) to make your system stronger. Cold water immersion encourages the clearance of old, worn-out mitochondria and stimulates new, healthy ones. The heat exposure of a sauna is linked to reduced inflammation and sends cellular messages, called 'heat shock proteins', that support collagen processing.

Avoid mitochondria enemies

- Don't smoke.
- Limit alcohol.
- Skip tanning and sunbeds.
- Avoid a sedentary lifestyle.

WHY IT'S NEVER TOO LATE

As we look to the future of skincare, it's easy to fall into the trap of thinking that the best results are reserved for those who started young. We hear that collagen begins to decline in our twenties, that sun damage accumulates silently, that prevention is everything. While these facts are sound, they're not the whole story.

The deeper truth – and the one I want you to take away from this book – is that skin remains biologically adaptable for your *entire* life. You do not get too old for progress. You do not miss the window. Even decades into adulthood, the skin can still build collagen, repair its barrier, refine its texture and brighten its tone. The science is clear: whether you start in your twenties or your sixties, well-chosen skincare can make a meaningful difference wherever you are in life. And it feels just as good when it happens.

If you start early, you're building strong foundations. If you start later, you're focusing on correction and optimization. Both paths lead to better skin. What matters most is consistency, clarity and choosing ingredients that truly deliver for your particular concerns.

This is why the future of skincare is so exciting. We're moving into an era in which evidence-based formulations, smart delivery systems and personalized routines empower *everyone*, at every age, to get results. The narrative is shifting from urgency and fear to agency and opportunity.

So, if there's one message I want you to take from this book, it's this: the best time to start is when you're ready. The next decade of your skin can be better than the last.

The future of skincare isn't about looking younger – it's about investing in your skin with intelligence, compassion and confidence. And no matter when you begin, your skin will respond.

ENDNOTES

2: SKIN 101

i Lyons AB, Moy L, Moy R and Tung R. 'Circadian Rhythm and the Skin: A Review of the Literature', *The Journal of Clinical and Aesthetic Dermatology*, September 2019; 12(9):42–5.

3: THE SKIN TYPE PREOCCUPATION

ii Cordain L, Lindeberg S, Hurtado M, Hill K, Eaton SB and Brand-Miller J. 'Acne vulgaris: a disease of Western civilization', *Archives of Dermatology*, December 2002; 138(12):1584–90. doi: 10.1001/archderm.138.12.1584.

iii Collier CN, Harper JC, Cafardi JA, Cantrell WC, Wang W, Foster KW and Elewski BE. 'The prevalence of acne in adults 20 years and older', *The Journal of the American Academy of Dermatology*, January 2008; 58(1):56–9. doi: 10.1016/j.jaad.2007.06.045.

iv Gether L, Overgaard LK, Egeberg A and Thyssen JP. 'Incidence and prevalence of rosacea: a systematic review and meta-analysis', *British Journal of Dermatology*, August 2018; 179(2):282–9. doi: 10.1111/bjd.16481.

v Duteil L, Queille-Roussel C, Lacour JP, Montaudié H and Passeron T. 'Short-term exposure to blue light emitted by electronic devices does not worsen melasma', *The Journal of the American Academy of Dermatology*, September 2020; 83(3):913–914. doi: 10.1016/j.jaad.2019.12.047.

5: DEMYSTIFYING ACTIVE INGREDIENTS

vi Bluemke A, Ring AP, Immeyer J, Hoff A, Eisenberg T, Gerwat W, Meyer F, Breitkreutz S, Klinger LM, Brandner JM, Sandig G, Seifert M, Segger D, Rippke F and Schweiger D. 'Multidirectional activity of bakuchiol against cellular mechanisms of facial ageing – Experimental evidence for a holistic treatment approach', *International Journal of Cosmetic Science*, June 2022; 44(3):377–93. doi: 10.1111/ics.12784.

6: BUILDING A SKINCARE ROUTINE

vii Bech-Thomsen N and Wulf HC. 'Sunbathers' application of sunscreen is probably inadequate to obtain the sun protection factor assigned to the preparation', *Photodermatology, Photoimmunology & Photomedicine*, December 1992; 9(6):242–4.

viii Narbutt J, Philipsen PA, Harrison GI, Morgan KA, Lawrence KP, Baczynska KA, Grys K, Rogowski-Tylman M, Olejniczak-Staruch I, Tewari A, Bell M, O'Connor C, Wulf HC, Lesiak A and Young AR. 'Sunscreen applied at ≥ 2 mg cm^{-2} during a sunny holiday prevents erythema, a biomarker of ultravioletradiation-induced DNA damage and suppression of acquired immunity', *British Journal of Dermatology*, March 2019; 180(3):604–14. doi:10.1111/bjd.17277.

9: THE FUTURE OF SKINCARE

ix Thau H, Gerjol BP, Hahn K, von Gudenberg RW, Knoedler L, Stallcup K, Emmert MY, Buhl T, Wyles SP, Tchkonia T, Tullius SG and Iske J. 'Senescence as a molecular target in skin aging and disease', Ageing Research Reviews, March 2025; 105:102686. doi: 10.1016/j.arr.2025.102686.

x Massudi H, Grant R, Braidy N, Guest J, Farnsworth B and Guillemin GJ. 'Age-associated changes in oxidative stress and NAD+ metabolism in human tissue', *PLoS One*, 2012; 7(7):e42357. doi: 10.1371/journal.pone.0042357.

All accessed 18 June 2026.

ACKNOWLEDGEMENTS

No book is written alone. While the words on these pages are mine, this book exists because of the generosity, wisdom, encouragement and belief of many people who have shaped both my thinking and my career.

To my agent, Viola Hayden, thank you for seeing the potential for this book long before it existed. Your belief in me, your guidance and your encouragement gave me the confidence to take on a project that often felt far bigger than I was. I am deeply grateful for your support and friendship throughout this journey.

To Ciara Finan, for stepping in these last months and helping carry the book over the finish line.

To Kate Fox, thank you for believing in this vision from the very beginning and for helping transform an idea into a reality. Your expertise, insight and guidance have been invaluable and this book is immeasurably better because of you.

To Juliette Norsworthy, thank you for all your assistance in making this book beautifully visual. You've helped to translate complex science into elegant, intuitive illustrations.

To Victoria Campbell, my friend, colleague and one of the smartest people I know. Your unwavering support, sound judgement and ability to see the bigger picture have shaped not only this book, but much of my recent professional life. There are very few people whose opinion I value as highly as yours.

To Jennifer Hoque, Creative Director at Dr Sam's, for casting your discerning eye over every illustration with patience and good humour always.

To my assistant, Dee Flaherty, and my team at Dr Sam's. You help me make my dreams come true every single day. Each customer review is a result of all your dedication and drive.

To Maria Boyle, thank you for understanding not only what I do, but why I do it. Your ability to challenge my thinking, tell me hard truths when necessary, and remain steadfastly supportive has made me better, and this book stronger.

To Professor Mark Birch-Machin, thank you for your generosity, curiosity and encouragement. Your pioneering work on mitochondria has profoundly influenced the way I think about skin health. Our conversations and collaborations exploring the role of cellular energy in skin health have inspired me enormously, and your support over the past few years has meant a great deal.

To the dermatologists who have trained me, challenged me and shaped the clinician I am today. I am indebted to Professor Nick Levell, Dr Clive Grattan, Dr Klaus Misch, Dr Portia Goldsmith, Professor Kieron Leslie, Dr Nisith Sheth, Dr Jacqueline Dyche, Dr Adam Friedmann, Dr Nemesha Desai, Dr Emma Wedgeworth, Dr Rakesh Patalay, Dr Emma Craythorne, Dr Rishika Sinha and Dr Mia Steyn. Medicine is a team sport, and I have been lucky in my teammates.

To Gill Gorman Round and Joanna Rogers – women I admire enormously in business, whose kindness, support and uncanny ability to impart the right wisdom at exactly the right time have helped me immensely as an entrepreneur.

To Sarah Jossel, who first came into my life as a patient and quickly became one of the earliest champions of both me and the brand. Your unshakable belief in my work and your friendship have meant more than you know. I have long admired your writing and your ability to cut through the noise with warmth, intelligence and lashings of common sense – qualities I have always aspired to bring to my own work.

To my patients, past and present, thank you for your trust. The questions you have asked, the stories you have shared and the challenges you have entrusted me with have taught me more than any textbook ever could. This book exists because of you, and I hope it serves you well.

To my incredible community, thank you for your trust, loyalty and belief in the mission. What began as a desire to help people better understand their skin has grown into something far bigger than I ever imagined. Nothing brings me greater joy than seeing someone gain confidence through mastering their skin. Thank you for allowing me to be part of that journey, and for believing, as I do, that when you change your skin, you can change your life.

And finally, to my family.

To my father, who taught me to dream big and pursue those dreams without fear, no matter how ambitious they seemed. You encouraged me to see possibilities where others saw limitations and gave me the confidence to follow my own path.

To my brother Shel, the hardest-working person I know. Your dedication to your craft has always inspired my own.

To my mother, who taught me the importance of kindness, generosity and believing in yourself. You never let practical constraints stand in the way of opportunity and always encouraged me to make the most of whatever life placed before me. Your love, support and staunch belief have shaped every part of who I am.

Whatever good comes from this book is rooted in the values my family has instilled in me. For that, I will be forever grateful.

INDEX

Dr Sam's

Dr Sam Bunting is a UK-trained medical doctor. She graduated from the University of Cambridge and University College London, and obtained her MRCP (UK) after three years of postgraduate medical training. She then completed seven years of intensive specialist training in medical dermatology and has over 15 years' experience in cosmetic dermatology.

She is the founder of Dr Sam Bunting + Associates at 41 Harley Street, and her eponymous skincare brand, Dr Sam's. She is known for her evidence-based, practical approach to skin health and for making expert skincare advice accessible. Through her media and TV work, including TLC's *Extreme Beauty Disasters*, Dr Sam helps demystify the beauty arena with clear, no-nonsense guidance.

@drsamsskincare

@drsamsskincare
@drsambunting

@DrSamBunting

Dr Sam's Skincare Club